Aesthetic Rhinoplasty

Aesthetic Rhinoplasty

Gilbert Aiach MD
Plastic and Aesthetic Surgeon, Paris
Attending Surgeon, Plastic Surgery Department,
Centre Hospitalier Universitaire Henri Mondor,
Faculté de Médicine, Paris

Jacques Levignac MD
Director of Post Graduate Education,
European Association for Cranio-Maxillo-Facial Surgery
Attending Surgeon, Department of ENT and
Maxillo-Facial Surgery, Hôpital Lariboisière, Paris

Forewords by
Paul Tessier MD
Former Head of the Department of Plastic Surgery,
Foch Hôpital Suresnes, Paris
Honorary Fellow of the American College of Surgeons
Doctor Honoris Causa, Lund University, Sweden

Georges Freyss MD
Professor of Oto-Rhino-Laryngology,
Head of the Department of ENT and Maxillo-Facial Surgery,
Hôpital Lariboisière, Paris

Translated by
S. Anthony Wolfe MD FACS
Clinical Professor of Plastic and Reconstructive Surgery,
University of Miami School of Medicine, Miami, Florida, USA

CHURCHILL LIVINGSTONE
EDINBURGH LONDON MELBOURNE NEW YORK AND TOKYO 1991

CHURCHILL LIVINGSTONE
Medical Division of Longman Group UK Limited

Distributed in the United States of America by Churchill
Livingstone Inc., 1560 Broadway, New York, N. Y. 10036,
and by associated companies, branches and representatives
throughout the world.

First English edition 1991

ISBN 0-443-04398-1

British Library Cataloguing in Publication Data
Aiach, G. (Gilbert)
    Aesthetic rhinoplasty.
    1. Man. Nose. Plastic surgery
    I. Title   II. Levignac, Jacques
    617.5230592

Library of Congress Cataloging in Publication Data
Aiach, Gilbert.
        [Rhinoplastie esthétique. English]
        Aesthetic rhinoplasty/G. Aiach, Jacques Levignac;
foreword by
    Paul Tessier, Georges Freyss; translated by S. Anthony
Wolfe. —
        1st ed.
            p.   cm.
        Translation of: La rhinoplastie esthétique.
        Includes bibliographical references and index.
        ISBN 0-443-04398-1
        1. Rhinoplasty. I. Lévignac, J.   II. Title.
    [DNLM: 1. Rhinoplasty. WV 312 A288r]
    RD119.5.N67A3513 1991
    617.5′230592—dc20
    DNLM/DLC
    for Library of Congress   90–15128
                                                   CIP

Aesthetic Rhinoplasty 2E, G. Aiach & J. Levignac
© Masson, Editeur, Paris, 1989

Produced by Longman Singapore Publishers (Pte) Ltd.
Printed in Singapore.

Foreword to the second French edition

This work is pleasing because it is practical and it is practical because it is simple. However, in spite of its small size, it is not a simplified version of a work on aesthetic rhinoplasty.

Rhinoplasty is not a technique, but a universe whose limits are far from being reached. All the galaxies and the stellar systems are found there in the form of phenotypes, morphotypes and types too often altered by inexperienced surgeons. The real talent of these authors has been to condense this universe into something useful in daily practice, instead of expanding into an encyclopaedic erudition. They have chosen from the innumerable procedures of which very few, since Joseph, have been original in spite of the tonnage of 'personal procedures', 'improvements' and 'refinements'. Their choice has been well made. Even better, this choice has been well applied and is well explained in the text, the drawings and the photographs.

One might say of this monograph that it is brief, that each type of nose is represented by only two cases or even one single case. This does not matter, since once evident success has been shown in a particular case, it can be reproduced. The accumulation of cases does not serve in its demonstration but, rather, becomes burdensome.

Of course, having seen the nose from all viewpoints, even through the cranial route, I would like to have found malformations, major traumatisms and nasal amputations. But this immense panoply would take us out of the area of aesthetic nasal surgery, which is large enough without having to extend into the greater but weightier area of facial orthomorphic surgery.

As it stands, this book will be useful not only to young surgeons but also to many experienced rhinoplastic surgeons, because the short case descriptions will remind them of valuable experiences which often become lost in the midst of our daily routines.

Paul Tessier

Foreword to the first French edition

This work dedicated to aesthetic rhinoplasty is useful, practical and well executed.

Unfortunately, more and more often, we see patients who are unhappy with the rhinoplasty they have undergone. One even sees true mutilations. Obviously, the consequences are then serious and the problems difficult to correct.

As is indicated in this work, rhinoplasty is a marvellous operation; but it must succeed at the first attempt. If all has been properly thought out and properly carried out, the result should have a 'natural' quality.

Of course one occasionally has to do a minor touch up procedure, in search of perfection. This is always what the patient is hoping for and what we aspire to.

If this work showed only the technique of rhinoplasty, it would be nothing new. It becomes original and particularly useful by going into difficult cases and the means of solving them. One gains from the experience of the two authors, with all the explanations one could want concerning the choice of procedure.

The results shown are convincing and prove their point. We should add that this work, in discussing the architecture of the nose, does not neglect nasal physiology. It does not pretend to be an encyclopaedia on the subject. But conceived as it is, we find it practical, easy to consult and, we feel, extremely useful.

It is a pleasure for us to recommend it.

George Freyss
Professor of Oto-Rhino-Laryngology
Hôpital Lariboisière, Paris.

Contents

Introduction

Why this work on rhinoplasty?

● First of all, because there are few works in the French language treating the subject completely and in detail. On the other hand, over the past few years there have been many interesting works which, taken together, have led us to re-think the problem.

● Secondly, because we feel that there has been a certain 'banalisation' associated with the increase in the number of rhinoplasties carried out, and this tends to make one forget how important the procedure is for the patient, and how deeply motivated he or she is to seek the operation. We should not forget that a rhinoplasty does not just change the nose; it changes the entire face because it alters its proportions. Knowing what the face means to an individual, the part that it plays in human relations, one can well understand how this 'simple' operation which has become so 'banal' can change a person's entire life. One then grasps the full measure of our responsibility.

We should recognise, before operating, that every error or misunderstanding can be serious. It is important to properly inform the patient at the outset as to what is possible and what is not, and to agree on a course of action.

What are we aiming for?

● Certainly, the problem is not purely one of geometry, and our approach is somewhat different to that adopted in the past, when certain surgeons always ended up with the same sort of nose which, in a way, was their signature. This is not what we are looking for! A nose well-operated on should not be noticed. Deeply aware of the beauty associated with differences that distinguish us one from another, and of the beauty in the difference, one should respect the personality of a face. This itself expresses morphologically in the overall relationship of the structures, the lines of the contours and the bony framework. We should note also that the problem in a woman, where the important thing is grace, differs from that in a man, where we would think that it is more one of 'character' emphasizing his strongest traits. One therefore plays on the nuances and the change of lines and proportions, doing away with caricature-like excesses and the unattractive aspects of a deformity.

● The most interesting thing, in fact, is not so much to change the nose, as to contribute, through changing it, by the removal of a negative aspect and the provision of a new harmony of the face, to an opening-up and blossoming of the personality. Rhinoplasty is thus seen as a determining act of 'surgical psychology'.

What is the order to follow?

● Firstly, one should carefully study the face in its three dimensions and also during movements of expression. Since the time of the ancient Greeks, there have existed rules which tend to establish what are accepted as ideal proportions; from this artistic research, inspired by philosophy, has come, over the course of time but particularly more recently, research related to dysfunctional anatomy which leads us to better understand the architecture of the face, the equilibrium of the forces at play, the integral movement of the form, postural phenomena and, associated with this last, the great cervicocephalic curvature.

The nose does not exist as an isolated entity; its projection occurs in relation to the forehead, as well in relation to the chin, and it is in this way

1

'that one positions it on the cervicocephalic profile. The face is naturally asymmetrical and there are true curves in the face. The nose follows these curves, and the movements of expression often accentuate asymmetry. All this should be seen, noted and analysed.

• Once the examination of the nose has been properly done, both the interior (to detect any anomaly, septal in particular), and the exterior (the nose in relation to the whole face), one establishes a course of action with the aid of photographs and, sometimes, xeroradiographs. This makes it possible to better explain to the patient what it is possible to do. There should not be any misunderstandings.

We turn now to the operation itself, and to the evolution of the technique.

• Concerning technique, it is our opinion that since Joseph invented rhinoplasty in 1928, there has been little major progress apart from that related to the study of procedures which are increasingly functional. In other words, one is not concerned with morphology alone, but, rather, ties together the two elements of form and function.

From this point of view, the technique of J. Andersen, called in France the dissection 'extra-muqueuse' (extra-mucosal approach), constitutes definite progress because it preserves the valvular function of the respiratory passage.

Cottle proposed a physiological rhinoplasty which respected the valve and also the integrity of the osteocartilaginous roof. This approach was well thought-out on a functional level, but we have found that there are serious limitations from an aesthetic point of view.

If the roof should be reconstituted, Anderson's technique facilitates the reimplantation of an altered hump as a free graft into a good recipient bed. More recently, more extensive anatomical and physiological studies have made it possible for us to better understand the mechanism of the nostril orifice, its role in respiration and also in expression; this leads one to avoid interfering with this mechanism, or at least to interfere with it as little as possible.

We will see, in fact, that a better understanding of the structures of the nose and of their physiological function, enables one to question a certain number of procedures or, for all practical purposes, eliminate them. Quite simply, one is able to do better work. Such an understanding defines and specifies what can and should be achieved.

A large number of procedures and ingenious 'tricks' have been described. We will explain those which in our hands have been the most useful.

• Instrumentation in rhinoplasty has always been of basic interest, and many authors have sought improvements. We will specify our instruments of choice.

• During the operation, the instrument is in the hand of the surgeon, which brings us to the operator, his plastic sense, his experience and his knowledge.

In certain hands, we have seen that, no matter what the technique employed, rhinoplasties almost always turn out well. Evidently, then, it is not the technique alone that counts. The plastic sense of the surgeon is at work from the beginning, dominating the operation and guiding it to the final model and towards success.

Is this plastic sense inborn?

We will leave the answer to this up to you. However, we will say, having looked at the results, that this sense seems to develop better in some than in others. Certainly, it can be cultivated. Rhinoplasty is, for those who perform it, very much a matter of taste, of judgement and of experience. Experience places the art in the context of what is possible, which is far from being the same in every case. It helps one to achieve the best possible result in each case, even though it is not the ideal. It makes it possible to provide what has been promised.

One needs to know everything about the subject, having been both warned and enriched by the experience of others. Let us explain what we mean by this:

In rhinoplasty, which consists of taking everything apart in order to put it back together again, difficulties during the procedure are not uncommon. Everything does not always go the way one would like it to. But with knowledge and experience, and with the 'little tricks' which we would like to give you, the surgeon can always get out of difficulty. One should always end up with a balanced nose which functions properly, is well proportioned and has the desired shape.

One should do what needs to be done! No more! No less!

The operation should be mentally rehearsed and every detail carefully calculated before it is embarked upon. If, by chance, a problem occurs during the procedure, this should be resolved in the course of the same operation. One of the objects of this book is to prepare the surgeon for the unexpected.

We propose that you *rethink rhinoplasty* through our experience, keeping clearly in mind what we owe to those who have preceded us. We apologize in advance for being unable to acknowledge every one, but we do not fail properly to describe the procedures which have been useful to us, and give the indications for their use. With respect, to this the presentation of the *selected cases*, along with photographs, analysis and drawings of the treatment are demonstrative and clear.

The chapter on 'Secondary rhinoplasty' is saved for the end and given particular attention. Three major types of complications stem from rhinoplasty, and the outcome of the operation should therefore be judged after about a year.

● Firstly, the rhinoplasty may be correctly performed, based on proper analysis, but it may be that nature is at fault due to abnormal scarring. It is good enough but nevertheless there remains a small defect: this is never particularly serious if the rules have been respected. The retouch will be easy. One can improve upon the improvement recently achieved, and thus arrive at the desired result.

● Secondly the operation may be conservative as far as the structural changes are concerned, but poorly conceived with respect to the relationship between the structures. The result is disappointing, and the rhinoplasty will have to be entirely redone. This will be more difficult, and the prognosis more cautious.

● Thirdly, the error may be greater: there may have been an excessive sacrifice of tissue which has led to deformity and functional impairment. One cannot correct the situation except with grafts. Very often, in these cases, the history is one in which a series of operations have been performed which have progressively aggravated the damage. Unfortunately, this is related to the phenomenon of 'banalisation' which we spoke about at the beginning. These cases are not rare.

It is important to understand that, for the patient who is hoping for so much from us and from this operation, this is a tragedy, and such a situation should be avoided at all costs. This is why we judge the chapter on 'Secondary rhinoplasty' to be so important.

As one understands these cases better, one learns how to avoid them and also how to get out of such difficulties.

The lesson we learn from complications is quite simple, it is also revealing: *A corrective rhinoplasty is an operation which should succeed the first time*. Properly carried out, it leads to a wonderfully natural result, and the old nose and the old face are immediately forgotten.

It remains for us now only to begin this rhinoplasty and to finish it with you; that is the aim of this work.

1. Surgical anatomy: Essentials of physiology

PART 1

SURGICAL ANATOMY

The nose has the form of a triangular pyramid, with its summit corresponding to the root of the nose and a base into which the two nostrils open. This pyramid (Fig. 1.1) has:

- Two lateral sides of varying obliqueness depending on the width of the posterior surface. The two lateral surfaces are made up of an osteocartilaginous expansion which joins at the midline with an osteocartilaginous expansion from the other side and with the anterior edge of the septum, which contributes to the solidity of the structure, to the support of the nasal bridge and

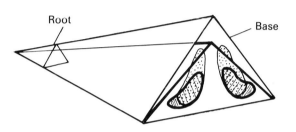

Fig. 1.1 Nasal pyramid.

to the projection of the nasal tip. This pyramid is thus an osteocartilaginous structure which constitutes the framework of the nose, and whose form is determined by:

— The form of the osteocartilaginous infrastructure

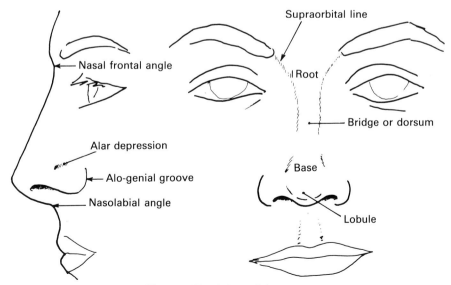

Fig. 1.2 Morphology of the nose.

5

— The thickness and the elasticity of the skin, the importance of which we will see later.

● The base of the nose has two nostril orifices, with the columella and membranous septum separating them. The columella continues into the lobule towards the tip of the nose. On each side, the nasal alae define the orifices which have a symmetry determined by the point of touchdown of the alar bases (Fig. 1.2).

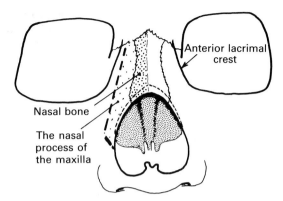

Fig. 1.3   Anatomical and surgical unit: nasal bone + nasal process of the maxilla.

THE NASAL BONY FRAMEWORK

Depending on the length of the nasal bones, the nasal bony framework occupies either the upper half or the upper third of the nasal framework; it is made up by the bones of the nose themselves and by the nasal processes of the maxilla.

1. The nasal process of the maxilla

— Joins superiorly with the medial orbital plate of the frontal bone and anteriorly with the nasal bone
— It has on its lateral surface the anterior lacrimal crest which forms the anterior limit of the lacrimal groove and represents the posterior limit of a lateral osteotomy line. It constitutes a palpable landmark.

2. The nasal bones (Figs. 1.3 and 1.4)

— They are constituted by two quadrangular plates which are vertically oriented.
— They are narrow and thick in their upper portion, and wider and thinner, in the lower part.
— Their superficial surface is smooth and concave in the upper half and convex in the lower half.
— Their medial border is very thick superiorly, thinner towards the bottom.
— Their lateral border, thinner, is bevelled at the expense of the superficial surface and articulates with the nasal process of the maxilla.
— The lower border is continuous with the triangular cartilage which is in fact covered by the lower border of the nasal bones; the union is accomplished by a thin conjunctival tissue which permits the triangular cartilage to be closely related to the nasal bone; thus violent manoeuvres, particularly

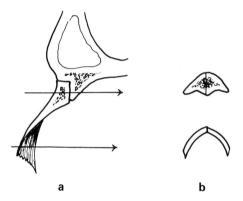

Fig. 1.4   a) Medial view of the nasal bone. b) Horizontal sections through the nasal bones.

with the rasp, can involve a partial disinsertion of the triangular cartilages.
— The terminal external branch of the internal nasal nerve emerges at the inferior border of the nasal bone after having passed along the deep surface of this bone where it leaves a groove which is more or less vertically oriented, and which is frequently mistaken for a fracture line on X-rays.
— The upper border of the nasal bone is thick, and articulates on each side with the medial orbital process of the frontal bone; it contributes, with the frontal bone, to the formation of a reinforcement and a zone of resistance at the level of the root of the nose.

3. The frontal bone shows at this level:

— The nasal indentation with an inferior convexity, and at its two extremities, the two medial orbital processes of the frontal bone.

— Posteriorly and in the midline, the nasal spine of the frontal bone, 10–20 mm in length, triangular, with a superior base whose rough anterior surface receives the crest formed by the coming together of the medial border of the two nasal bones.

— The posterior surface of the nasal spine of the frontal bone, corresponds to the superior portion of the anterior border of the perpendicular plate of the ethmoid. In most cases, the high fracture after a lateral osteotomy takes place at the junction of the thick and thin portions of the nasal bones. In hypertrophies involving the nasal root, a resection can create a high disarticulation of the naso-frontal suture.

— To the osseous vault, formed by the nasal bones, extends and joins a median septum constituted here by the perpendicular plate of the ethmoid.

THE MIDDLE THIRD. THE SEPTUM

Often more projecting, corresponding to the *cartilaginous framework*, the middle third of the nose is more supple but still contributes to the solidity of the entire framework and, in particular, makes it possible to explain the suppleness and the mobility

of the nose; a suppleness and mobility which increases further at the level of the nasal tip.

At the level of the middle third are located the triangular or (upper lateral) cartilages.

1. The triangular or upper lateral cartilages have (Figs. 1.5 and 1.6)

A medial border which fuses with the lateral expansions of the anterior septal border in its upper two-thirds. In the lower third, they are separated from the septum which facilitates inward and out-

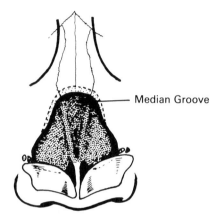

Median Groove

Fig. 1.5 Triangular or upper lateral cartilage.

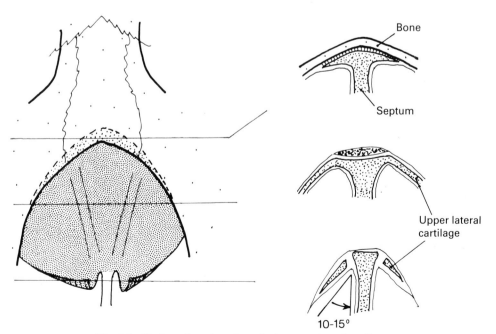

Bone

Septum

Upper lateral cartilage

10-15°

Fig. 1.6 Horizontal sections through the upper lateral cartilages.

ward movements of the cartilage during nasal respiration.

A median groove, visible after removal of the perichondrium, marks the limit between the triangular cartilages and the lateral dorsal processes of the anterior septal border.

A superior border which is in relationship with the inferior border of the nasal bones; the attachment takes place by a dense fibrous tissue at a height of 2–10 mm which decreases from inward to outward (Fig. 1.6).

At the level of the superior portion of the piriform orifice, the periosteum is in continuity with the perichondrium which surrounds the triangular cartilage.

An inferior border which extends from the piriform orifice to the septum; it slides under the lateral crus of the alar cartilage to which it is joined by a dense tissue, a prolongation of the superficial and deep perichondrial layers in which are located several fragments of cartilage called 'sesamoids'. These fragments are partially excised during the operative procedure (Fig. 1.7).

This portion is often folded back on itself over 2–3 mm like the collar of a shirt.

2. The muscular and aponeurotic system

The triangular cartilages and the alar cartilages are at the centre of a *muscular and aponeurotic system* which includes (Fig. 1.8):

A superficial portion muscular and aponeurotic, which extends over the entire nasal pyramid and attaches below to the superior border of the alar cartilages, covers them, and then extends into the deep surface of the dermis.

A deep portion, which is the continuation of the periosteum from the piriform orifice, the periosteum blending into the perichondrial layer which surrounds each portion of cartilage.

The triangular cartilages are of major importance in nasal physiology; their medial borders should, after a rhinoplasty, have anatomic relationships which are close to normal if one wants to preserve satisfactory function.

3. The cartilaginous septum

The cartilaginous septum or quadrangular cartilage (Fig. 1.9), is an anterior extension of the bony septum; its shape is roughly quadrangular; it passes under the cartilaginous roof.

The septal cartilage has:

An antero-superior border which contributes to the shape of the cartilaginous bridge:

● In its upper third, this border is located under the deep surface of the nasal bones.

● In its middle third, it is in close relationship to the upper lateral cartilages: the anterior septal border enlarges to form two lateral expansions which articulate with the medial borders of the upper lateral cartilages through a dense fibrous

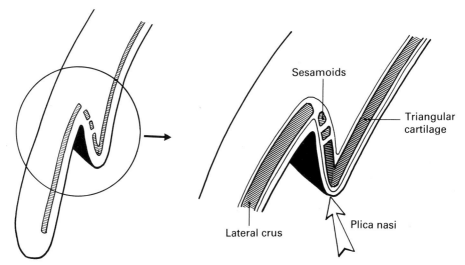

Fig. 1.7   Sagittal section in the midportion of the nasal ala.

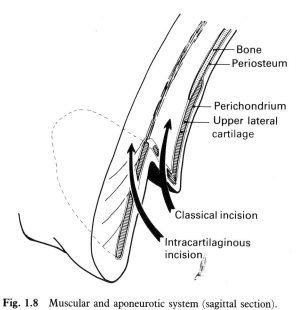

Fig. 1.8 Muscular and aponeurotic system (sagittal section).

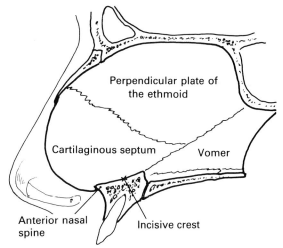

Fig. 1.9 The septal framework.

articulation. The anterior border of the septum is wide superiorly and narrows from above downward.

● The lower third is separated from the superior cartilages and is clearly behind the cartilaginous domes (about 1 cm), an anatomic separation which one should be able to note at the end of the operation.

There is there a zone of soft tissue (the triangle of Converse), which can be the location of a temporary hypertrophy after the operation (Fig. 1.10).

An antero-inferior border, extending obliquely posterior, forms a rounded angle with the antero-superior border; it rejoins the nasal spine to which it is firmly bound by a perichondrial and periosteal tissue which extends around at this level to constitute a tight but rather mobile articulation.

A postero-superior border, joined to the perpendicular plate of the ethmoid by a tight attachment, but which can show itself to be fragile during a harvesting of these two pieces in continuity.

A postero-inferior border, extending obliquely from posterior to anterior; this flared border narrows posteriorly and has a caudal prolongation which extends between the ethmoid and the vomer.

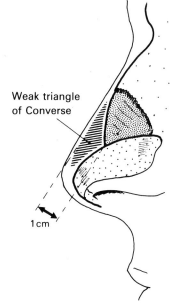

Fig. 1.10 Weak triangle of Converse.

Anteriorly, the inferior border expands to install itself on the incisive crest which sometimes becomes a groove to hold this border. Often, however, the inferior border slides over one of the flat lips of this groove and then projects to one side with a corresponding respiratory obstruction.

The union with the incisive crest takes place through perichondreal and periosteal fibres which permit a certain mobility of the septum.

The septal cartilage contributes in an important fashion to the projection of the tip of the nose, through its antero-superior border. By its narrow connections with the upper lateral cartilages, it assures the support of the middle third of the nasal pyramid, which plays an active role in nasal respiration.

It is important to understand properly the morphology of the cartilaginous septum, particularly the articulations of its postero-superior borders with the perpendicular plate of the ethmoid, and the postero-inferior border with the vomer, because these articulations both contribute to the stability of the septum, and also are often involved during corrective surgery for malformations of the septum, and during harvesting of the septum as a graft, since the septum constitutes an important and very useful donor source; the amount of material that can be harvested makes it possible in certain cases to avoid harvesting an iliac graft.

The ideal location for harvesting a large osteo-cartilaginous graft is along the inferior border of the quadrangular cartilage, a little behind the nasal spine which is preserved, and extending down back to the posterior border of the vomer.

The harvesting can be of cartilage alone or can be osteocartilaginous.

THE LOWER THIRD AND THE ALAR CARTILAGES

The lower third comprises the supple and mobile portion of the nose. The nasal tip is supported by the alar cartilages which determine its shape.

The alar cartilages have the form of an arch composed of (Fig. 1.11).

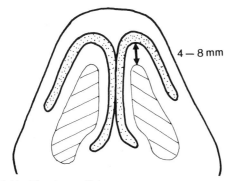

Fig. 1.11 The alar cartilage.

1. The mesial crura

The two mesial crura come together at the midline where they take part in forming the columella; habitually straight, the mesial crura can undergo deformities partly related to a deviation of the inferior septal border. Furthermore, it is not rare to discover, during the dissection of the dome, one mesial crus which is shorter than and differs from the other, without this being in evidence on external examination.

The posterior ends of the mesial crura diverge and can sometimes involve a marked enlargement of the base of columella. This enlargement is often caused by a prominent nasal spine which extends between the foot plates of the mesial crura.

At the level of the nasal tip or lobule, the mesial crura diverge to form the dome and then the lateral crura.

2. The lateral crura

The lateral crura are quadrangular and usually convex (Fig. 1.12).

Their length varies from 17 to 30 mm with a mean of 22 mm the lateral end or the posterior prolongation extending down to the edge of the piriform orifice; this posterior prolongation has the form of a delicate neck more or less divided into cartilaginous islets.

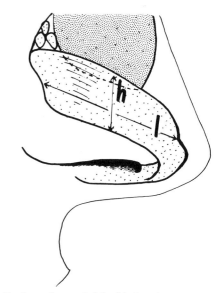

Fig. 1.12 Lateral crus: height (h), length across (l).

The height of the lateral crura varies from 7–15 mm, with a mean of 11 mm. The superior border of the lateral crus covers superficially the infero-lateral border of the triangular cartilage which is often curved back upon itself. The articulation between these two pieces takes place through the deep portion of the musculo-aponeurotic and fibrous system which joins these two structures.

The manner of these connections also explains why the nose does not lengthen with age; in fact, this lengthening, which occurs only slightly or not at all in individuals having a small nose, is seen particularly in large noses: it is caused by relaxation of the tissue due to the weight of the surface skin.

The inferior border of the lateral crus does not follow the alar rim (Fig. 1.12):

— Near the dome, the distance is 4–8 mm (mean 6 mm)
— In the middle portion, it is 3–7 mm (mean 5 mm)
— In its lateral and posterior portion, from 9 to 19 mm (mean 13 mm)

The inferior border thus extends upward posteriorly sometimes in an important fashion. It is possible to see the projection of this inferior border in individuals with thin skin when the cartilages are rigid: posterior pressure on the tip of the nose causes a projection of the inferior border of the dome which blanches the skin; an endonasal examination makes it possible to locate the inferior border of the lateral crus when one elevates slightly the inferior nostril border.

The variations of the lateral crura are numerous and diverse; they have been classified by Zelnick as:

— smooth convex
— convexed anteriorly, concave posteriorly
— concave anteriorly, convex posteriorly
— concave anteriorly and posteriorly with a convexity in the intermediate portion
— concave over its entire length.

Symmetry is not always evident in spite of an apparent symmetry of the nasal tip; certain concave portions can be filled in by soft tissue of varying thickness.

3. The dome

The dome is located at the union of the lateral and medial crura; near the tip or the lobule, the lateral crus has a sudden narrowing which constitutes the lateral extent of the dome.

The domes are of quite variable shape and form a curve of varying openness, sometimes very pinched and sometimes quite broad.

Their lower border is at some distance from the nostril border. This space is made up of the superposition of the external and vestibular skin.

Any marginal incision should extend along the inferior border of the cartilage.

Among the variations which can involve the alar cartilages and the triangular cartilages, besides variations in shape, there exist variations in thickness, rigidity and suppleness of the cartilages; one can determine this by palpating the tip of the nose. This examination provides important information which can affect the operative considerations. Certain nasal tips are quite firm, have a good spring, whereas others are soft and without consistency and seem to have no support.

THE 'PLICA NASI' AREA (Figs. 1.7 and 1.8)

The plica nasi is made up of the lower edge of the triangular cartilage which abuts on its deep surface with the superior border of the lateral crus and constitutes an anatomical landmark; the incision is usually located below the plica nasi, which is to say through the lateral crus. The classical high incision, in the plica nasi, leads to a deeper plane of dissection, in contact with the triangular cartilages, whereas a lower, intracartilaginous incision, leads to a plane of dissection which is more superficial and passes through the muscular and aponeurotic system.

The choice of plane of dissection should therefore be determined in part by the thickness of the nose.

SOFT TISSUES OF THE NOSE

This plays a very important role in rhinoplasty. It is, in effect, a skin of varying thickness which covers the osseous and cartilaginous structures and determines to a certain extent the shape and the fineness of the nose, in particular of the nasal tip.

Three distinct zones can be established according to the thickness and connections of the cutaneous layer.

In the upper third, the skin is of moderate thickness; in fact, it has a thick layer of fat and muscular tissue which permits considerable mobility in the area of the nasal frontal angle.

In the middle third, the skin is thinner but very mobile over the osseous portion from which it is separated by a musculo-aponeurotic layer by a thin layer of weak cellular tissue. This mobility diminishes considerably toward the tip.

In the lower third, the skin becomes thicker, rich in sebaceous glands, with pores open to varying degrees, particularly at the level of the lobule and the nasal alae.

It is also very adherent to the underlying structures of muscle and cartilage. It is this greater thickness which limits the ability of the skin to retract after the reduction of the alar cartilages.

The thickness of the skin covering this osteo-cartilaginous skeleton can be appreciated with precision on a lateral xeroradiogram where one can note the marked thinning in the middle portion of the nose (see xeroradiographic study, page 18).

ORIFICIAL MUSCULATURE AND PIRIFORM ORIFICE

We will study the muscles which cover the bony framework and the cartilaginous support structures, which fix to them, and — attaching also to the cutaneous layer and causing its movements — participate in facial expression. They are:

— *Superiorly*, the *pyramidal muscle*, the *transversus muscle*, the *superior levator muscle* of the nasal ala and the upper lip, and the *dilator* of the nasal ala (Fig. 1.13).
— *Inferiorly*, the fan-shaped (*myrtiform*) muscle and the *depressor of the nasal septum*.

In fact, the anatomical description which one can give, and which varies in different textbooks, only makes sense after a study of their function, which helps us to understand the synergies and antagonisms at play, that is to say the functional equilibrium of a region where the orbicular muscle of the lips also has a determining role, not forgetting also the other muscles of facial expression.

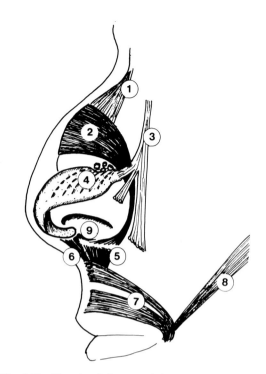

Fig. 1.13 Functional diagram of the musculature ① pyramidal; ② transverse; ③ superficial levator of the nasal ala and the upper lip (several fibres connect it to the transverse muscle); ④ dilator of the nasal ala; ⑤ myrtiform. The lateral fibres are in continuity with the upper fibres of the transverse muscle; ⑥ depressor septi nasi; ⑦ orbicularis of the lip: the upper fibres are oblique and pass over the depressor septi nasi (in this particular case); the lower fibres are horizontal; ⑧ zygomatic: it attaches to the skin and to the mucosa of the upper lip; ⑨ nasal spine.

The musculature of the nose itself, we should state at the outset, has an important role in regulating the flow of air in breathing. There is an evident relation between the muscles which extend around the piriform orifice and the dimensions of this orifice. The *nasal index* is described by the formula:

$$\frac{\text{Maximum width} \times 100}{\text{Maximum height}}$$

The variations of the nasal index, studied throughout the evolution of man, and as a function of adaptation to climate, are revealing, extending from the *leptorrhine* of the Eskimos (where one can note the predominance of the 'constrictor' system of the nostrils in a very cold climate), to the *platyr-*

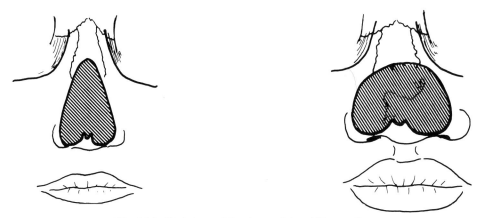

Fig. 1.14 Variations of the shape of the piriform orifice.

rhine of the negroes of Gabon (where, in contrast, the width of the piriform orifice signifies the predominance of a dilator system) (Fig. 1.14).

Form follows function, and the nose is an essential organ of adaption to climate.

The chapter on anatomy aims to emphasize the importance of the orifice mechanism, which is to say the entirety of the muscles and cartilage of the tip, because while the cartilage supports the tip, it is the muscle which animates it (J. Levignac, J. C. Chalaye, E. Mahe and R. Riu). To do this, we will study in turn the anatomy and the physiology of this region. Of the many works available on the respiratory physiology of the nose, very few deal with the mechanism of the orifice.

In the seven methods used for this investigation, two seem to us essential: *microdissections* and electromyelographic study.

MICRODISSECTIONS

These provide two types of essential information:

1. They confirm the existence of a subcutaneous, premuscular, musculo-aponeurotic layer, which has blood vessels in it and is exactly comparable to a SMAS, whose lower portion is attached to the upper part of the alar cartilages, explaining the absence of a sliding plane at the level of the nasal tip. It is this layer, (more than the thickness of the skin) which reduces the visibility of the cartilaginous junctions.

2. They provide important information on the descriptive and topographical anatomy of the muscles. Thus, in our study, the dilator of the nasal ala appeared absolutely constant (J. C. Chalaye, Fig. 1.13).

It is a very delicate fan-shaped muscle, with an inferior tip that extends between the antero-inferior portion of the alar cartilage, anteriorly, and the antero-inferior portion of the upper lateral cartilage posteriorly; the tip extends between the two cartilages where it mingles with the outer fosciculus of the myrtiform or fan-shaped muscle, the medial fibres of the transversus and the infero-medial fibres of the common levator [we will see later, thanks to EMG studies, that this muscle has no connection with the adjacent muscles (unlike the others)].

If one accepts the postulate of the cycle, nerve–muscle–chondro–osseous development, it appears that it is the dilator of the nasal ala which is responsible for the projection of the nasal ala, because it is the only muscle which inserts entirely on the nasal ala; it is a muscle which is much more developed in the black race.

The common levator has a well-developed nasal fasciculus, which inserts on the infero-lateral portion of the nasal ala and on the perichondrium of the alar cartilage (this fasciculus is necessarily removed during resections involving the nostril attachments).

The transversus passes over the nasal ala and has narrow connections with the common levator and the outer fasciculus of the myrtiform at the level of the piriform orifice; then, by its infero-medial fibres, it rejoins the region of the nasal

anterior-inferior nasal spine. Since it is the same on both sides, we have here the equivalent of an 'orbicularis' of the nose. Our own study and analysis emphasized this, as did the study of J. Delaire in 1978.

The myrtiform is a vertical muscle having the form of a fan with an inferior base. Its superior fibres reach vertically to the anterior floor of the nasal fossae, the lateral fibres have a relationship with the transversus and the common levator, and the medial fibres have connections with the depressor of the nasal septum and the superior fasciculus of the orbicularis.

The depressor of the nasal septum or depressor septi nasi extends between the anterior portion of the dome and the anterior surface of the nasal spine, in front of the mesial crura and behind the superior fascicle of the superior orbicularis, like a cord of an arc; this explains why, during laughter, the orbicularis of the upper lip contracts and pulls posteriorly the depressor of the nasal septum. The tip of the nose is then pulled posteriorly and downwards (Fig. 1.15).

With respect to this last description, it should be mentioned that there is a close relationship between the orifice system of the nose and the orbicularis system of the lips and that the point of convergence of the two systems is the region of the antero-inferior nasal spine (J. C. Chalaye).

ELECTROMYOGRAPHIC STUDIES (EMG)

In addition to this anatomical study, electromyographic studies have brought us important information on the physiology of the nasal orifice which is indispensable to understand the mechanism of constriction and that of dilatation.

The common levator. Its essential action is to open up the nasal ala. It is a dilator, increasing the nostril orifice in its transverse sense. Its function becomes more important during exertion.

The transversus. This is a powerful constrictor, and an accessory dilator by its lateral fibres.

The proper dilator. This is a dilator only, and is not involved in constriction; it has a not unimportant action during speech as well as a permanent tonic activity associated with the respiratory cycles.

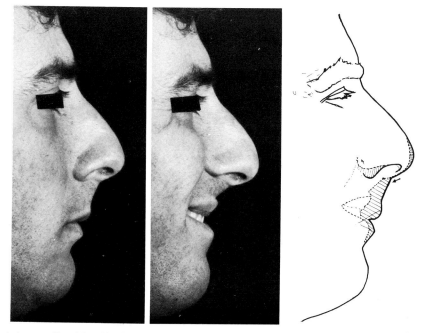

Fig. 1.15 Suspended upper lip with projecting nasal spine. The peripheral fascicles of the orbicularis are elevated and form a band during smiling, pulling on the depressor septi nasi; (under the action of the zygomatic muscle, the tip of the nose is pulled backward and slightly inferiorly).

The myrtiform. One can distinguish: lateral fasciculi which are primarily constrictor. A weak EMG response to dilatation seems to us associated with the muscular equilibrium and to the play of the antagonistic muscles.

The medial fasciculi of the myrtiform are essentially constrictors. The more one nears the midline, the more the EMG response to dilatation weakens.

The muscles, by a valvular action which is constantly in play and involves the cartilages, determine the shape of the nostril orifices and therefore the form of the entire nasal tip: if the projection of the tip of the nose is generally inversely related to the spreading out of the base, it depends above all on the spring of the alar cartilages. The muscles of the nostril floor (the myrtiform and some of the transverse fibres) maintain the effect of the spring.

In this study, we should mention in passing, a working hypothesis: that there exists in the face, receptors, both thermal and baroreceptors, whose role is to inform the central nervous system on the conditions of the environment, and that these centres in turn order the constriction or the dilatation of the nostril orifices, a phenomenon of adaptation to the initial phases of respiration.

The localization of these receptors as well as their histochemical nature and their afferent pathways is being studied; the efferent pathways necessarily involve the facial nerve, because it is the only nerve enervating the muscles of the nose. . .

In conclusion:

— It appears to us essential to understand the relationships between form and function.

— To want to understand the important role of the muscles in morphogenesis does not go against genetics and its laws which explain the resemblances seen in the same line, and also the extraordinary variety of forms associated with different combinations.

— We should know that besides the orifice and respiratory mechanism that directs these muscles, the latter participate in another manner which is also very essential, in the acts of facial expression, which is under an action which equilibrates with the other muscles of the face.

In conclusion. Practical surgical considerations involving rhinoplasty:

1. We recommend great prudence during surgery surrounding the nostril passages. The indications are limited. There have been nasty and unpleasant complications.

If one carries out this surgery with an aesthetic aim, in an African for example, one condemns this person either to live in a temperate climate, or to become a mouth breather in his own country because one removes or reduces his powers of adaptation.

2. In the choice of technique, our preferences end toward those that:
— take account of physiological data, including that during exertion
— respect the orifice mechanism and particularly the dilator system, because it is most often threatened during rhinoplasties
— do not alter expression, the nostrils being in their movements very revealing of emotional life, of sensibility and of sensuality.

3. It appears to us worthwhile to propose electromyographic study of the nasal muscles in certain common ventilatory abnormalities, including those which are sequelae of rhinoplasty.

RHINOPLASTY: THE STEPS OF ANATOMICAL RECONSTITUTION

It is above all at the level of the nasal dorsum that it is interesting to study the anatomic modifications that follow the resection of a hump and the performance of 'lateral osteotomies'.

The resection of the osteocartilaginous hump creates a nose which appears to be wide and flat, which necessitates a lateral osteotomy on each side to bring together the lateral portions of the nose, i.e. the two osteocartilaginous flaps, and thus to close the bony roof.

The osteocartilaginous flap

After a resection of the hump and lateral osteotomy, the osteocartilaginous flap becomes an individualised **anatomic unit** (Fig. 1.16).

It is made up of:

A superior osseous portion which results from the close union between what remains of the nasal

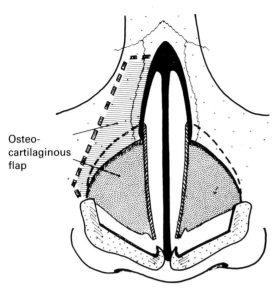

Osteo-
cartilaginous
flap

Fig. 1.16   The osteocartilaginous flap: An anatomical and surgical unit.

bones and the nasal process of the maxilla, separated from the maxilla posteriorly by the lateral osteotomy.

The cartilaginous portion is made up of the upper lateral cartilage whose anterior or medial border has become free because of the section of the lateral dorsal prolongations of the anterior septal border. These osseous and cartilaginous portions are connected by dense connective tissue, but this connection, in the form of an overlapping, occurs over a length which becomes even shorter as the resection of the hump becomes greater, leading to a certain fragility which is accentuated by traumatic manoeuvres such as the violent use of the rasp.

The osteocartilaginous flap has:

— A completely free *anterior border* which after the osteotomy and in fracture should move medially; but because of the variable convexity of the lateral wall of the nose, only the inferior cartilaginous portions and the most superior osseous portion are particularly close to the midline.
— A *posterior or lateral border* which corresponds to the lateral osteotomy line
— A *free inferior border*
— A thick *superior border* which corresponds to the fracture line resulting from the outward lux-

ation (out-fracture) or the inward luxation (in fracture) of the osteocartilaginous flap after the osteotomy. This fracture line is often incomplete, like a greenstick fracture, and this can contribute to the limitation of the mobility of the osteocartilaginous flap.

The *superficial surface* of the osteocartilaginous flap can be divided into two portions: one medial where the skin has been undermined; the other lateral, where the skin should remain adherent.

The *deep surfaces* are covered by nasal mucosa which, because of the extramucosal dissection, has not been sectioned, and extends from the septum to this deep surface, then continues on to the lateral wall of the nasal passage.

Thus, this rectangular osteocartilaginous flap has, after the osteotomy, a certain mobility which depends in part on its surface. The shorter the bone is, the more the flap which is predominantly cartilaginous is at risk of falling into the nasal passage; this becomes more likely to happen when the lateral osteotomy is too anterior, as this reduces the width of the flap.

THE NASAL TIP SUPPORT

The nasal tip support has two elements which are (Fig. 1.17a):

— Firstly the framework of the alar cartilages, whose form, thickness, and consistency can vary from one case to the other, but whose suppleness explains the fact that during trauma, for example, the support of the tip of the nose sustains relatively little damage. One can encounter adherent or fragile cartilages with the stigmata of old trauma which are manifested by tearing more easily than normally, but this damage is much less than that observed on the septum or on the bony bridge.

The action of the two mesial crura which are leaning against one another can be compared to that of a tent pole which extends down to the ground, which is in this case, the nasal spine; this explains why an excessive resection of the nasal spine can be associated with a loss of the nasal tip projection.

— The second element of the nasal tip support is constituted by the cartilaginous bridge (dorsum) which contributes to the support of the skin

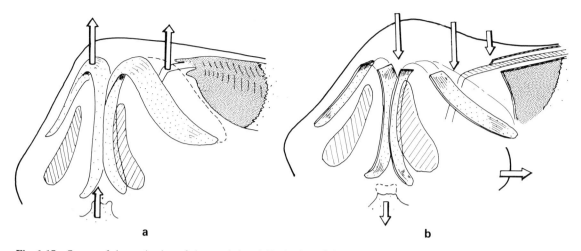

Fig. 1.17 Causes of the projection of the nasal tip. **a)** Projection of the nasal tip is assured by: the domes, the cartilaginous bridge (dorsum); the nasal spine. **b)** Lowering of the nasal tip is caused by: lowering of the bridge, reduction of the height of the domes and the lateral crura; resection of the domes; resection of the nasal spine; a transfixion incision extended to the nasal spine; thick skin, and weak cartilage.

framework which is itself adherent to the alar cartilages.

Lowering or weakening of the septum can bring about a diminution of the projection of the tip of the nose, particularly when the nose is broad and flattened and when the cartilages are lacking in spring.

Reinsertion or a graft at the level of the cartilaginous bridge can bring about, at the same time that it augments the projection of the bridge, an effective projection of the tip with a discreet lowering or rotation of the structure inferiorly.

The surgical manoeuvres which can bring about a loss of the nasal tip projection are therefore (Fig. 1.17b):

— An intersepto-columellar incision which is extended posteriorly
— Lowering of the septal bridge (resection of the osteocartilaginous hump)
— Resection of the cartilaginous domes— Resection of the cephalic excess of the lateral crura
— Resection of the posterior extensions of the lateral crura
— Resection of the nasal spine.

This loss of nasal tip projection will be much more noticeable and marked in wide, flattened noses with thick skin, than in narrow noses with a long columella.

XERORADIOGRAPHY IN THE STUDY OF THE DEFORMITY

In the preoperative study of the nasal profile, a lateral X-ray with a soft beam or a xeroradiogram can be useful for the study of the soft tissues and the osteocartilaginous profile.

At the level of the naso-frontal angle, the thickness of the soft tissues reaches its maximum near the nasion (this precise landmark corresponds to the anterior extremity of the naso-frontal suture). This thickness varies between 3 and 9.5 mm; these are the extremes, and the majority of cases fall between 7 and 7.5 mm (7 mm in a female and 7.5 mm in a male) (Fig. 1.18).

At the level of the upper portion of the nasal hump or the rhinion, the thickness of the soft tissues is reduced considerably, to a mean of only 2 mm (extremes of 1 or 3 mm).

● The naso-frontal curve: This is not regular, but it can be represented in general by a circle drawn in the osseous naso-frontal concavity.

● The outline of the osseous and cartilaginous profile:

— The osseous profile line is carried from the most posterior portion of the osseous concavity (situated at the level of the nasion or 1–2 mm below) to the summit of the osseous convexity located at the most inferior portion of the nasal

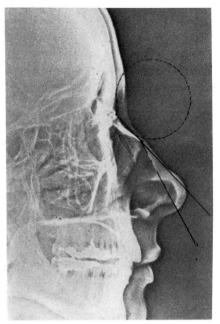

Fig. 1.18   Lateral xeroradiograph. Osseous and cartilaginous profile lines.

bone, this later point being located several millimeters above the rhinion (the most anterior point of the osteocartilaginous junction)
— The cartilaginous profile line is sometimes clean and straight, which facilitates the tracing, but it is sometimes less clean or convex; in this case, it is represented by a tangent to the summit of this convexity;
— These two osseous and cartilaginous profile lines form an angle which varies from one case to the next.

Practical conclusions from those constructions

— The osseous naso-frontal curve has a diameter which is smaller when:

● the glabella is more projecting
● the osseous hump is more prominent.

— The thickness of the soft tissues increases when the diameter is small, that is, when the osseous depression is more marked.
— The study of the variations of the angle determined by these osseous and cartilaginous profile lines is more interesting; this angle is:

● open with prominent osseous humps; this is why, when one resects the hump with an osteotome, the direction of the instrument should be modified according to the direction of the cartilaginous section, which varies from one case to another.
● less when the bridge is straight or concaved.

PART 2
PHYSIOLOGICAL DATA AND FLOW REGULATION
R. Riu

The nose is the organ of smell, as we all know. But it also plays an essential role in respiratory regulation which deserves some attention.

1. The function of the nose are:

— to regulate the volume of air in relation to the thoracic bellows
— to filter the air
— to warm the air
— to humidify the air.

2. This is accomplished by a double mechanism:

Internal. This mechanism involves essentially the pituitary mucosa and the valve of the turbinate. The alternation of congestive phenomena between one nasal fossa and the other, with a periodicity of three hours on average, means that overall nasal resistance does not change and that this cycle is not perceptible (R. Riu).
The external orifice. This involves the *vestibular valve*. Its effects are influenced by the muscles which surround it.

There are, in fact, three vestibular narrowings which are, from front to rear:

— the external nostril orifice, having an area of about 1 cm^2
— the internal nostril orifice, limited laterally by the plica nasi, and medially by the septum, at the level of the zone of transition between the cuta-

neous and the mucosal epithelium. Its surface areas is about 1.25 cm^2.

— the nasal isthmus of Bachman or internal ostium of Zukerkandl, or nasal valve of Mink. This narrowing is the true vestibular valve or nasal valve.

Elaborate rhinorheographic techniques have established the sites of resistance in the nasal fossa, and have replaced the classical notion of a valve including the plica nasi and the septum, with that of the region of the nasal valve limited (Fig. 1.19):

— Laterally, by the limen nasi, a mobile shape formed by the plica nasi and the soft tissues connecting the alar cartilage to the piriform orifice.
— Medially, by a septal line obtained by the projection of a plane perpendicular to the septum, at the level of the limen nasi.

— At its lower portion, by the inferior border of the piriform orifice.
— At its upper portion, it forms an angle of 10–15° which varies according to the air pressure and the muscular adjustment. It corresponds to the indentation of the lower one-third of the septo-triangular junction filled in by a fibrous tissue. This is the membranous valve. The valve is triangular in shape, with an inferior base and a surface area of about 0.7 cm^2.
— If with respect to the surface anatomy, one can distinguish the internal nostril orifice, the true internal border of the vestibule of the valve, a portion partly including the nasal fossae.
— The nasal pyramid is differentiated into the fixed nose and the mobile nose, the hinge of which is situated at the level of the membranous septo-triangular indentation, a true joint of the

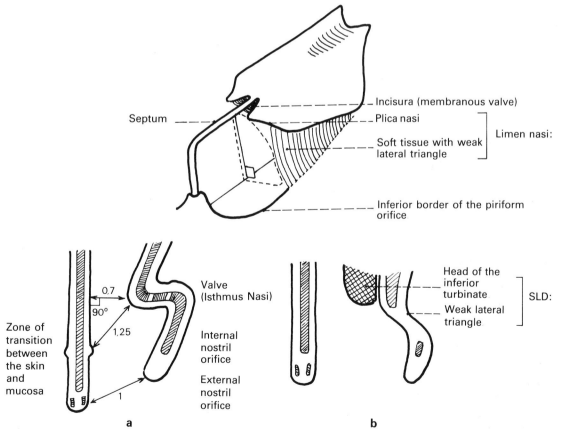

Fig. 1.19 The Valvular system. **a)** Section through the plica nasi. **b)** Section through the inferior portion of the limen nasi.

cartilaginous roof (Wayoff-Tisserant) playing a primary role in the dynamics of the valve.

— The triangulo-alar junction, having intimate connections through the intermediary of the cartilaginous plates enclosed in a single perichondrial sheath (Jost), does not therefore have the role of the joint which is usually attributed to it.

The lower border of the cartilage has an outward concavity, and the lateral crus of the alar cartilage has an internal convexity. Thus, there is formed an anatomical arrangement preventing the valve from collapsing and establishing a force which is opposed to that provided by the upper two-thirds of the triangulo-septal junction: The septal T.

On the other hand, a physiological tendency separates the inferior border of the upper lateral cartilages from the septum, at the level of the incisura, preventing the collapse of the valve during inspiration. This concept of a functional unit of the valve and the ala of the nose is important.

The valve has an adjustable convergent-divergent form permitting the inspiratory and expiratory passage of a volume of air one and one-half times greater than that which would pass during the same period of time if the nasal fossa had a simple orifice without narrowing.

The lateral wall of the valve, which is supple, is particularly mobile inferiorly at the level of the junction of the lateral crus. During normal, light inspiration, the lateral wall is depressed and there is a slight closing of the valve inferiorly. During a deep inspiration, this closure is more marked.

During a forced inspiration, the voluntary contraction of the dilator muscles prevents closure and, if necessary, opens the valve. The function of the valve, in relation to the musculature, increases the respiratory delivery according to need. The valve controls, orients and changes the inward flow of air through the nostril, which narrows at the level of the valve and is able to involve the greatest surface area of mucosa, the more so since the valve of the turbinate creates turbulences which further favour contact between the airflow and mucosa. The filtration, humidification and regulation of the temperature of inspired air are thus facilitated.

It should be recognized that a certain degree of nasal resistance (NR) is necessary and physiologi-cal. It depends on the calibre of the nasal fossae and on the volume or rate of the respiratory flow, and is expressed in cm water. Overall nasal resistance (NR) varies between 0.8 and 2 cm water. If it goes beyond 2 cm water, the valve dilates, and at about 4 cm water the valve closes and mouth breathing begins.

The collapse of the valve is due to particularity of the limen nasi, which has a segment limiting the nasal delivery of air (SLND). This depressible segment acts in such a way as to increase the nasal resistance in proportion to the flow, which thus remains constant. The SLND controls therefore the respiratory flow, and prevents damage to the inferior air passages during certain circumstances (exertion, stress) which increase the air flux to a considerable extent.

The SLND is formed by two elements: the head of the turbinate becomes filled with blood and increases nasal resistance in proportion to the delivery of air, and at the same time it produces a collapse at the level of the weak upper lateral cartilage situated between the inferior border of the triangular cartilage, the nasal process of the maxilla and the postero-superior border of the ala, at the level of the cauda. This collapse is also proportionate to the airflow. When the flow increases, the SLND tends to move toward the external nostril orifice. There exists, therefore, a true valvular system.

In certain narrow noses, where there is a vasomotor rhinitis, or more often in certain sequelae of rhinoplasty, the SLND collapses more easily, with the appearance of secretions which create what we call the 'syndrome of the wet nose'.

This depressible segment does not exist in blacks. This is one of the reasons for the greater physical endurance of blacks, whose mechanisms of conditioning inspired air are more developed. The SLND can, therefore, be considered a physiological handicap.

During the congestive phase of the nasal cycle, the valve of the turbinate predominates in NR.

In the phase of vasoconstriction, it is the vestibular valve. Nasal respiration takes place preferentially on the non-congested side. This shows the importance of the vestibular valve.

Injuries to the valve cause an interference with respiration on exertion, and are marked by an abnormal increase of NR in certain conditions which concern us. A disinsertion of the upper lateral cartilage, an excessive luxation of one of the bones can interfere with the function of the limen nasi. An excessive resection of the lateral crus alters the functional solidarity of the alar valve of the nose. For the same reasons, reductions of the ala of the nose should be parsimonious and exclusively cutaneous.

On the other hand, correct rhinoplastic incisions rarely disturb the solidarity of the alar valve of the nose, because they are located in the region of the triangulo-alar junction which is not a true articulation. There are no functional differences between inter- and intracartilaginous incisions, because the resections at the level of the triangular cartilages and the alar cartilages are carried out after the incision made to the cicatritial consolidation at the level of the triangulo-alar junction. The vestibular stenoses are due to incisions with overly generous resections.

During rhinoplasty, certain surgical manoeuvres can have a beneficial effect on the play of the valve.

Anomalies of the inferior border of the upper lateral cartilage should be corrected by a prudent resection, whether the anomaly consists of a thickening, an irregularity or an excessive rolling up. The striations intended to break an abnormal nasal spring are illusory, considering the lack of thickness of the cartilage; either they are ineffective because they are too superficial, or else they go all the way through the cartilage and break it up, which is not satisfactory.

In order to conserve the lateral movements of the valve, it is desirable, after resection of the inferior border of the upper lateral cartilage, to reproduce the physiological indentation of the septum by resecting a small triangle with an inferior base, whose summit rejoins the septal cartilage.

Sometimes, due to an upper lateral cartilage which is a bit short, a simple incision is adequate.

A septal deviation in the region of the valve should be corrected by repositioning the septum, rather than by a resection which creates an additional depressible segment.

A hypertrophy of the head of the turbinate should be treated by cauterisation if it is mucosal, or by turbinectomy if it is osseous.

Finally, in narrow noses, or in those affected by a vasomotor rhinitis, a cauterisation of the head of the inferior turbinates continuing into the limen, at the level of the depressible segment, adjacent to a weak lateral triangle, and associated with a resection of the inferior border of the piriform orifice by a buccal approach, can serve as a preventative treatment of the syndrome of the postoperative wet nose.

These surgical gestures are facilitated by the extramucosal approach.

PART 3
PREOPERATIVE ANALYSIS AND PLANNING OF THE CORRECTION

Preoperative studies should not be limited to an examination of the nose.

All corrective surgery requires an extended *psychological examination* which should precede the general examination. The affect, psychological state and motivations of the patient should be studied with care, because they can have a very considerable effect upon the decision on whether to operate or not.

In the general history, besides the usual contraindications for surgery, one should check particularly about a history of allergy, a tendency to bleeding, ecchymosis, and the formation of bad scars.

1. The nose as a part of the face

Artistic anatomy is concerned not only with the nose but also and particularly with its relationships with the other parts of the face with which harmony should be achieved. We search for the 'golden number', which draws our attention to the relationships of the parts both between one another, and with the whole. The forms and the curves, the shape of the forehead, the movement and position of the upper lip, the prominence of the cheekbones, the bone structure of the face, all influence us in carrying out the correction.

Within the nose itself, there are masses which may or may not be in equilibrium. This is the case with the nasal tip and the nasal bridge; a large nasal tip seems less voluminous if the bridge is augmented by a cartilaginous or osseous graft.

We thus see that:

— The projection of the nasal bridge can be more or less noticeable according to whether the forehead is flat or curved, whether the naso-frontal angle is prominent or hollow and, particularly, whether the chin is prominent or receding.

— A slight naso-maxillary osseous hypoplasia with a naso-genial depression can make the nose seem more projecting.

— Sometimes, a prominent appearance of the eyeballs is accentuated by an exaggerated flattening of the nasal bridge.

— When the nasal bridge is hollowed or flattened, the eyes appear further apart.

— A long upper lip is partially masked if there is a long nose and in this case it is thus contraindicated to overly shorten the nose.

— On the other hand, a lower third of the face which is short benefits from the shortening of a nose which is too long, as this accentuates the mouth or the upper lip.

— As a rule, the naso-labial angle is more often open (100–110°) in women. Consequently, shortening the nose can feminise it, and care should be taken when the patient is a man.

2 Examination of the nose itself

An external examination should be carried out (frontal, lateral, and worms eye view), together with a rhinoscopic examination and an examination of respiratory function.

Besides a careful inspection, the nose should be palpated in order to study the skin, the junction of the triangular cartilages of the bone, and the resistance of the alar cartilages and of the nasal tip.

• *The frontal examination* should take note of:
— asymmetry: deviation of the nose or facial asymmetry
— the width of the bridge and the nasal tip
— the length of the nose
— the appearance of the alae, a difference in their level, and the extent of nostril exposure.

• *The examination in profile.* It is usually for the correction of the profile that the patient comes for a consultation, most often for a kyphosis or a bony or cartilaginous predominance, the magnitude of which should be assessed in relation to the projec-

tion of the tip of the nose and the naso-frontal indentation, but also to the curvature of the face.

At the level of the tip of the nose, one should note, besides the projection, the relationship of the alar margins with the columella, the naso-labial angle, the columellar-apical angle, the length of the nasal alae and, finally, modifications which take place at the tip of the nose during facial expression — retraction and downward displacement.

• *Oblique view.* This should be done from the left and right; this is important, because an osseous projection is sometimes only noticeable from one side.

• *The examination of the nostril orifices with the head extended* makes it possible to note asymmetry of the columella, often associated with a subluxation of the lower septal border, but also the appearance of the nostril orifices, the nasal alae and the foot of the columella.

• *Examination of the internal valve* can be done by simple observation of the movements of the valve during inspiration, where one can check that the valve retracts with inspiration, without a collapse which interferes with respiration.

• *The condition of the skin* plays primary role and the patient should be informed of the important contribution of the type of skin to the result obtained, particularly when the skin is thick and fatty.

Rhinoscopy, with the aid of a headlight, is indispensable during the examination, because if a septal deviation exists, it should be corrected *in the same operative session* as the aesthetic correction.

One studies:

• *The appearance of the nasal mucosa*, sometimes pale, and other times congested.

• *The possibility of a deviation.* A posterior deviation without an effect on nasal morphology or an anterior deviation which can have an effect on the bridge; the appearance of the inferior turbinates which are sometimes hypertrophied, violacious, or oedematous and washed-out, suggesting a nasal allergy.

• *The appearance of the plica nasi, the suppleness of the internal valve* and the angle formed by the upper lateral cartilage with the septum which should be 10–15° (Fig. 1.16).

All this data should be noted on an appropriate form, partly in the form of a diagram.

3. Photographs

Photographs, (front, lateral and inferior view, on a 13 × 18 cm format) are necessary, not only to give the patient an idea about his future appearance, but also so that, once operated upon, the patient can see himself as he was 'before'.

It is useful, and above all practical, to put the account of its operation on the back of the profile photograph, partly in the form of a diagram showing at life-size the extent of the resections or the grafts carried out.

PART 4
ANAESTHESIA

A rhinoplasty can be carried out under *general anaesthesia,* with an endotracheal intubation, or under *local anaesthesia.*

The type of anaesthesia varies from one surgeon to another and often from one country to another.

General anaesthesia ensures the operative comfort of the patient and of the surgeon. It is preferred by many. Bleeding is perhaps greater than with local anaesthesia, and here the role of the anaesthetist is particularly important; he has manoeuvres which can reduce bleeding to a tolerable level.

As for local anaesthesia, it is often used in combination with powerful analgesic and narcoleptic drugs which induce a certain indifference and absence of memory in certain patients. With this, one often approaches general anaesthesia.

In fact, the only cases where one can operate in tranquillity using local anaesthesia without supplementation and without the presence of an anaesthetist, are those limited to a discreet retouch.

1. General anaesthesia

1. 15 minutes before the procedure, a *nasal packing* is placed (gauze 5 cm wide, soaked in xylocaine-naphthazoline). These packs are placed on the length of the nostril floor, against the turbinates and under the osteocartilaginous roof. This causes vaso-constriction, and therefore a reduction of bleeding, a better look inside the nasal passages, and a shorter operating time.

2. Then, *endotracheal intubation* — with the tube coming out in a midline position — and packing with prosthetic gauze or cotton.

3. A *local infiltration,* with saline or a 0.5% of xylocaine-adrenaline solution should precede the operation. This provides several advantages:

— a lighter general anaesthesia
— reduced bleeding
— a preparation of the planes of dissection.

The infiltration is carried out between the skin of the osteocartilaginous skeleton, trying not to overly deform the nasal bridge and the tip of the nose, and is carried out submucosally. It aims to block the sensory innervation.

At the end of the infiltration, gentle pressure is carried out for 1–2 min to spread around in a homogeneous fashion most of the injected solution, thereby reducing the external deformity.

The anaesthetist should keep in mind our needs and requirements during general anaesthesia.

2. Local anaesthesia and the distribution of the sensory nerves (Fig. 1.20).

The infiltration begins at several elective points taking account of the origin of the nerves, their appearance in the operative area, then of their distribution along the outer surface of the nasal pyramid, in the nasal fossae and on the septum. A brief review of the anatomy is therefore given below:

The nerves

Sensory enervation is provided by the trigeminal nerve. In particular:

1. The ophthalmic nerve (VI) This gives off the nasal nerve which itself divides into:

— An external nasal nerve, for the skin in the root of the nose;

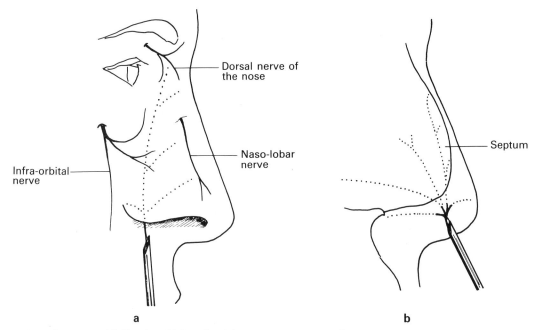

Fig. 1.20 a) Latero-nasal infiltration. b) Septal and intersepto-columellar infiltration.

— An internal nasal nerve, which penetrates through the anterior ethmoidal foramen and divides into two branches:
- one medial, destined for the anterior portion of the septum
- the other external, or 'naso-lobar' which, passing along a groove in the posterior surface of the nasal bone, innervates the skin of the lobule.

2. *The superior maxillary nerve* (V2) This is the most involved nerve. It emerges at the infra-orbital foramen and distributes several branches toward the nasal processes of the maxilla, but beforehand, at the very base of the pterygo-maxillary fossa, it gives off the *spheno-palatine nerve*. The latter divides into:

— The superior nasal nerves, fine branches which pass through the spheno-palatine foramen into the nasal fossae, and are distributed to the upper and medial turbinates
— The naso-palatine nerve which also passes through the spheno-palatine foramen into the nasal fossae, reaching the septum where it descends and gives off its branches, ending by passing through the anterior palatine foramen.
— The anterior palatine nerve, which descends laterally in the posterior palatine canal and distributes its branches to the mucosa of the soft palate, and also to the inferior turbinate.

This study of innervation, while showing it to be somewhat complex, also indicates the points of attack for local anaesthesia.

In summary

To summarise, the following are necessary:

- Firstly, 15 minutes before the operation, topical anaesthesia at the level of the spheno-palatine nerve and its branches, just behind the tail of the middle turbinate. This is essential for the entire lateral wall of the nasal fossae and turbinates.
- Packing is immediately followed by a preliminary 'diamond shaped' infiltration involving a cutaneous injection at the level of the root of the nose and an intra-oral injection at the level of the nasal spine (Fig. 1.21). These two injections are less painful than the endonasal injections which are carried out 15 minutes later when they are almost painless.
- The intranasal infiltration itself uses 0.5% xylocaine with adrenaline. One should not exceed 20 cm^3 in total.

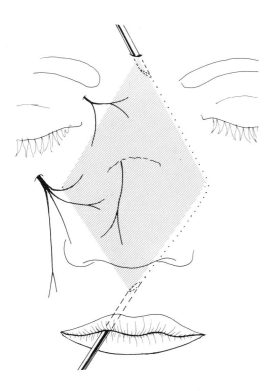

Fig. 1.21 'Losenge'-shaped anaesthetic infiltration carried out from the naso-frontal angle and the inferior nasal spine.

One infiltrates:

— Through the vestibular nasal mucosa (Fig. 1.20a):
    a. towards the infraorbital foramen
    b. along the line of the osteotomy,
    c. at the level of the alar foot plate;

— Next, towards the root of the nose, along the bridge and the tip. (One lightly injects along the inferior border of the nasal bone, where the naso-lobar nerve emerges)

— Then, in the intrasepto-columellar space, from the tip towards the nasal spine (Fig. 1.20)

— One carries out an infiltration of the septal mucosa going as far possible superiorly and posteriorly to reach the branches of the medial nasal nerve and the naso-palatine nerve. It should be noted that the physiological interruption of the latter shows itself also in the upper incisor teeth. This infiltration carried out down to the nasal floor will facilitate the subsequent submucosal and extramucosal dissection.

We should note, finally, that the discovery of new drugs which are tranquillising or even briefly anaesthetising (Ketamine), but of short duration, increases interest in local anaesthesia.

2. Technique

Rhinoplasty was invented entirely by J. Joseph. This inspired idea is easy to describe. It consists of first isolating the osteocartilaginous skeleton from its skin coverage by means of an endonasal incision, which leaves no visible trace, and then modifying these structures to the dimensions and proportions which are desired. The skin, because of its natural elasticity, follows the new shape of the underlying structure.

However, a rhinoplasty is an operation in which merely to possess the surgical technique is not enough to obtain good results. Each patient has a different nose and it is essential to adapt the technique according to not only the other facial characteristics but also to factors such as personality.

The aim of the operation is to obtain a nose which is as natural as possible, and which does not look like an item placed in the middle of the face. This leads to conservative surgery which has a double advantage; the physical aspect is improved without being excessively transformed, and the secondary defects are less frequent than when resections have been excessive.

We will describe here the three successive stages in a rhinoplasty.

1. Surgery of the tip
2. Lowering of the profile line
3. Narrowing and reconstruction of the dorsum.

However, it may be no less logical or indicated to begin by lowering the profile line. It depends on the case and this will be explained below.

In any event, each stage is carried out taking into account the modifications which are envisaged during the other stages; each portion of the nose should be considered as intimately related to the others; this applies above all to the relationship between the width of the bridge and that of the tip, and that between the height of the profile line and the projection of the tip of the nose.

INCISION LINES

The initial incision of a rhinoplasty has two portions which should be very precisely located. It is preferable to carry this out in three stages.

1. The intersepto-columellar incision

This can be *partial* or *total* (Figs. 2.1 and 2.2); it should be located at the *inferior border* of the septum and preserve the membranous septum which is left attached to the columella.

The membranous septum is the result of the coming together of the two septal mucosas beneath the inferior septal border. This assures the mobility of the columella relative to the septum. Its sacrifice therefore risks reducing the mobility of the lower portion of the nose.

The lower border of the septum is far from the medial crura at the tip and it is almost in contact with them posteriorly. The intersepto-columellar incision (transfixing incision), which should follow the inferior septal border, should avoid cutting into the septum posteriorly.

A double hook is placed at the summit of the nostril orifices; two single hooks are placed symmetrically on each side of the base of the columella and, pull it downwards, permitting a completely symmetrical transfixion incision. The latter is carried out after locating the lower border of the septum by use of a blunt instrument, such as the end of the scalpel handle.

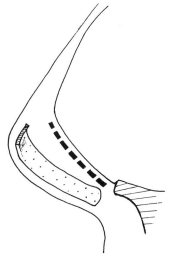

Figs. 2.1 and 2.2   Intersepto-columellar incision.

Fig. 2.1

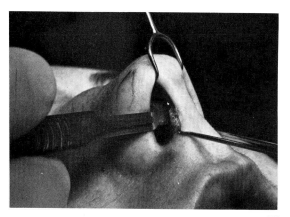

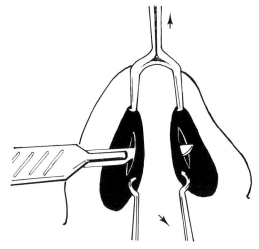

Fig. 2.2

This incision (Fig. 2.3) can if indicated, be extended down to the nasal spine, either using the scalpel, or with scissors, eventually permitting complete mobility of the skin relative to the underlying osteocartilaginous framework. One should avoid carrying the incision towards the nostril sill, as this risks the formation of a retractile band at this level.

However, if the naso-labial angle does not require modification, and particularly if no shortening is necessary, it is preferable not to carry the intersepto-columella incision too far.

2. The lateral incision (Fig. 2.4)

This can be into the mucosa only, facilitated in this by the infiltration of the vestibular skin; this

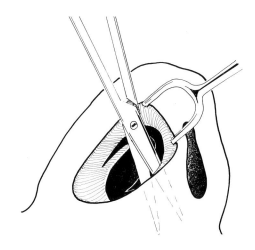

Fig. 2.3   Dissection carried towards the nasal spine.

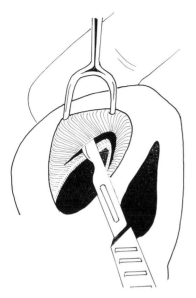

Fig. 2.4 Lateral incision.

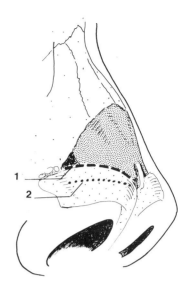

Fig. 2.5 Lateral incision: **1.** intercartilaginous incision; **2.** intracartilaginous incision.

permits the removal in one piece of the cartilaginous excess of the lateral crus so that it can be reinserted if required. It is simpler to section at the same time the cartilage whose upper excess will be removed later.

The location of the incision is classically intercartilaginous, but one may prefer an intracartilaginous incision for two reasons (Fig. 2.5):

— The first is that the alar cartilage always extends superficially beyond the inferior border of the upper lateral cartilage which forms the 'plica nasi', the site of the internal valve whose integrity should be conserved because of its importance in nasal respiration.
— The second reason is that the lateral crus is often quite high, which leads to an overly high incision. The latter should not therefore take account of the height of the cartilage, but, rather, of other factors, such as the ease of access possible through the nostril orifices, the difficulty of surgery of the tip, the importance of the resection of the excess of the lateral crus, and the suppleness of the skin.

A double hook is placed under the nostril border, and external digital counter pressure is used to immobilise and make the zone of the incision projecting (Fig. 2.4). The incision is carried out

from above downward, to the posterior limit of the subperiosteal dissection which will be carried out at the next stage. It extends posteriorly and should straighten out vertically if one wants to avoid breaching the posterior extension of the lateral crus which should be respected.

● Millard and Peck recommend a low intracartilaginous incision, parallel to the lower border of the lateral crus and situated about 3–5 mm from this border. The advantage of this is to permit at the same time the excision of the superior excess of the lateral crus, and to have a good exposure particularly in small or narrow nostrils and in thick skinned noses where eversion is difficult.

● One carries the incision into the intermediate section which corresponds to the region of the dome; carrying out this incision the three stages makes it possible to be more precise (Fig. 2.6).

UNDERMINING OF THE DORSUM

The beginning of the undermining can be carried out with a scalpel (Fig. 2.7), the depth of the incision depending on the thickness of the skin; if the skin is thin, the scalpel blade passes flush against the upper lateral cartilages. If the skin is thick, one can leave a layer of fatty tissue on the

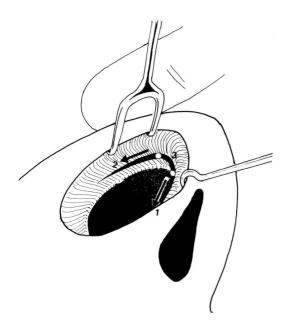

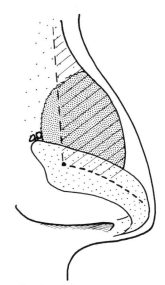

Fig. 2.8 Zone of undermining.

Fig. 2.6 Making the incision in three stages:
1. intersepto-columellar; **2.** lateral; **3.** at the level of the dome.

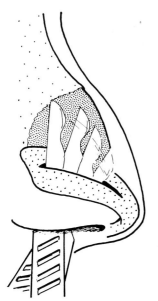

Fig. 2.7 Subcutaneous undermining begun with the scalpel.

outer surface of the upper lateral cartilages; this layer is then removed later (Fig. 2.7).

The width of the undermining depends on the width of the nasal bridge, the extent of the proposed recession of the bridge, and also on the extent of shortening. It is evident that a short nose with a discreet hump requires only limited undermining, whereas a long nose with a marked kyphosis requires more extensive undermining (Fig. 2.8).

The aim of the undermining is to separate the cutaneous cover from the osteocartilaginous skeleton on which the resections will be carried out; but also to permit the skin to adapt, thanks to its elasticity, to the new osteocartilaginous infrastructure.

1. The subcutaneous dissection

This is used in large hypertrophic noses with thick skin, in old nasal fractures, and in the area of the naso-frontal angle if it needs to be hollowed out. In the latter case, the cutting edge of the elevator sections the muscle fibres of the pyramidal muscle in the upper portion, and brings these fibres inferiorly in order to remove them with the osseous resection.

Laterally, the lateral cutting surface of the periosteal elevator is used to section the periosteum so that the nasal hump which is excised will be completely free.

The thickness of the cutaneous cover determines the extent of the incision of the fatty tissue.

2. Subperiosteal undermining

This is the most frequently used approach, particularly in noses with thin skin. It makes it possible to preserve a certain thickness:

- to assure a better curvature
- to mask small irregularities
- to soften the contours
- to better adapt the tissues to the new bony framework.

The intracartilaginous incision having been made, the undermining is begun with a scalpel at the outer surface of the upper lateral cartilages up to the inferior border of the nasal bone. The planes of dissection of the two sides are joined together. The undermining is then carried out by a Joseph elevator. After the periosteal incision at the lower border of the nasal bones, the elevator resting in contact with the bone is passed up laterally to the posterior limit of the undermining (Fig. 2.9 [1]); then, in a similar way, it is completed towards the midline with downward movement of the medial edge of the instrument, to connect up with the undermining carried out initially over the outer surface of the upper lateral cartilage (Fig. 2.9 [2]).

The upper edge of the periosteal elevator sections the periosteum at the root of the nose (Fig. 2.9 [3]). In this way one avoids forcing the periosteum upwards.

If the undermining has been carefully carried out, excision of the hump will be easy to perform.

The undermining can be carried down to the tip of the nose by using a curved button hook scalpel which makes it possible to keep the plane of dissection in continuity with the interseptocolumellar transfixing incision (Fig. 2.9 [4]).

At the end of this stage:

One should verify the absence of residual adherences between the skeleton and the soft tissues, and excise under direct vision the fragments of fatty tissue.

If there is significant bleeding, one should place a small compress soaked in saline solution in the space that has been undermined, and exert pressure for one or two minutes.

After the undermining, it is preferable to carry out shortening if it is indicated; this permits a

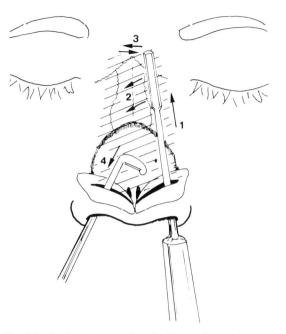

Fig. 2.9 Undermining continued with a periosteal elevator (**1, 2, 3**) and completed with a curved button knife (**4**).

greater ease of elevation of the skin cover by the use of an Aufricht retractor.

INTERNAL SUBPERICHONDRIAL, SUBMUCOSAL AND SUBPERIOSTEAL DISSECTION IN THE 'EXTRAMUCOSAL' DISSECTION
(Fig. 2.10)

The 'extramucosal' dissection is an important preliminary step:

— For the resection of the osteocartilaginous hump without tearing the mucosa
— For the correction of a septal deviation, a correction which is easier because of the preliminary septal lowering.

The other advantages of this extramucosal dissection are:

— The anatomical character of the dissection, which respects the mucosa and thereby respiratory function
— Less bleeding
— A postoperative course which is simpler both in the usual rhinoplasties and in those with bone

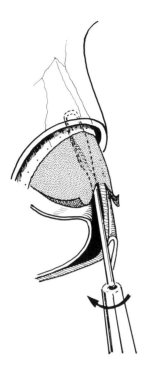

Fig. 2.10 Extramucosal dissection: the mucosal dome is separated from the osteocartilaginous dihedron.

— The inferior border of the upper lateral cartilage sometimes curved like a 'U', which will be excised (Fig. 2.11). The lower border of the upper lateral cartilage is then clearly identified. An S-shaped retractor elevates the nostril border, a forceps with teeth is placed over the inferior border of the mucosal dome, that is, on the inferior free border of the mucosal dihedron. After having carried out the shortening if this is indicated, the sub-perichondrial undermining is begun at the antero-inferior border of the septum along the entire length of this border and over a vertical distance of 0.5–1 cm, which makes it possible to excise more easily the excess cartilage, to arrive at the nasal spine much more easily and, finally, to facilitate the suturing at the time of closure.

The subperichondrial undermining is carried along the anterior septal border by tunnelisation, the Joseph elevator progressing slowly up to the root of the nose; then, the lateral edge of the periosteal elevator is used to carry out an inward turning movement which permits the liberation of the mucosal dome and the undermining of the mucosal lining of the osteocartilaginous roof for several millimeters (Fig. 2.10). The mucosa is

or cartilage grafts where the graft is located in a closed compartment and therefore has less risk of elimination and rejection.

J. Anderson was the first to properly describe this method, which permits the osteocartilaginous resections to be done while at the same time conserving the integrity of the nasal mucosa. J. C. Robin first introduced the technique to France.

TECHNIQUE

A preliminary submucosal infiltration at the level of the inferior septal border and at the level of the anterior dihedron makes the dissection quicker and easier.

The extramucosal dissection is preceded by an operative stage consisting of a 'stripping' of the superficial surfaces of the upper lateral cartilages over which one can find:

— Fragments of cartilage corresponding to the upper portion of the lateral crura
— Remaining fatty and muscular tissues

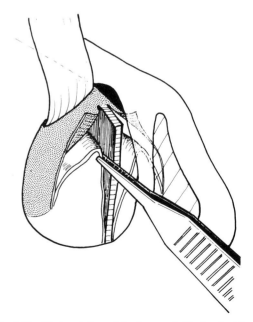

Fig. 2.11 Undermining of the 'mucosal dihedron' with an elevator.

much more adherent to the deep surface of the upper lateral cartilages, where it is thinner and more fragile, and it is often useful to infiltrate along the anterior borders of the upper lateral cartilages, in order to facilitate the undermining, which can be completed inferiorly with sharp scissors. The same manoeuvre as carried out on the other side.

At the end of this dissection, one should be able to perfectly distinguish on each side the mucosal dome separated from the osteocartilaginous reflection.

When the recession of the osteocartilaginous bridge is large, the mucosal domes can project between the osteocartilaginous incisions. This can be avoided, by undermining the mucosa a little further on the septal side and laterally, to permit it to fall back. If this is insufficient, or if the bridge of the mucosal dihedron is very thick, one may thin it by prudent excision with scissors, without piercing the superficial layer of the mucosa.

An associated septal deviation can make it necessary to continue the undermining from the lower border of the septum and the maxillary crest, down to the nostril floor. The septal undermining, however, may not join up with the anterior tunnelisation of the extramucosal dissection if the deviation is low or posterior.

SHORTENING OF THE NOSE

Shortening of the nose should take account of:

— The length of the nose and its appearance in frontal view
— The appearance of the naso-labial angle
— The columellar-apical angle
— The length and the appearance of the upper lip
— The appearance of the bridge: the existence of a hump, a straight bridge, or a saddle deformity.

In the male, an angle of 90° is desirable, whereas in the female this angle can be more open (100–110°), but it is evident that the appearance of the mouth (the upper lip in particular) and of the chin should be studied before carrying out the shortening.

Shortening is carried out on the lateral walls and on the septum in the midline. It should be quite prudent and moderate, particularly as far as the mucosa is concerned. It is much more difficult to lengthen a short nose than it is to shorten a nose which has remained a bit too long.

1. Shortening of the septum

This should be moderate, because it is surprising to see how small an excision is necessary to obtain the desired effect.

A useful and simple manoeuvre consists of drawing on the index finger, with its pulp resting in the naso-frontal indentation, an ink mark opposite a reference point drawn on the tip of the nose; then, elevating the tip of the nose to the desired level, another mark is made on the finger. The distance between these two marks makes it possible to evaluate the extent of shortening (Aufricht test: Fig. 2.12).

The resection along the inferior septal border can be (Fig. 2.13):

a. Either triangular, with a posterior summit, removing en bloc a fragment of cartilage covered with mucosa on both surfaces; this shortening has an effect of raising the tip of the nose while the upper lip *remains unchanged*. It can be performed with a scalpel which sections the mucosa and cartilage at the same time, describing an open angle, the advantage of which is to avoid a straight appearance to the columella (Fig. 2.14). Sometimes, the shortening is very anterior, making it possible to elevate the tip alone and not the nostrils.

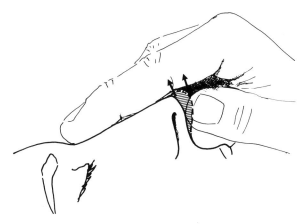

Fig. 2.12 The Aufricht test. A mark on the index finger indicates the length of the nose; the nose is shortened by pressure with the thumb, and a second mark is made on the index finger; this indicates the shortening required.

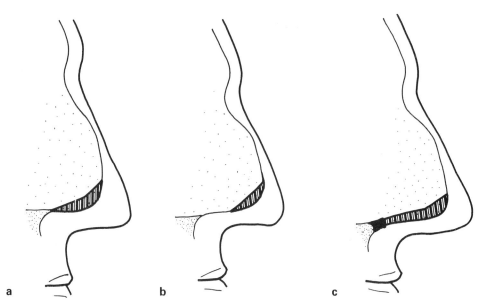

Fig. 2.13 Shortening **a)** triangular (long nose with normal upper lip); **b)** anterior triangular (raises only the tip); **c)** rectangular (long nose with short upper lip). The shortening encroaches on the inferior portion of the nasal spine.

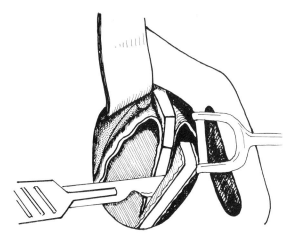

Fig. 2.14 Triangular shortening by resection of cartilage and mucosa en bloc.

b. Or rectangular, which permits a complete elevation of the columella, with a consequent increase in the length of the upper lip, a reduction in the length of the nose without a modification of the naso-labial angle.

2. Correction of a naso-labial projection

This can be carried out at the same time as the shortening: in fact, the naso-labial angle can be very open because of an excessive projection of a hypertrophic nasal spine. The nasal spine pushes the soft tissues forward, elevates the lip and the orbicularis and causes an enlargement of the foot of the columella.

One can initially extend the intrasepto-columellar incision towards the nasal spine which one then strips on its two surfaces and on its inferior border with a periosteal elevator.

The reduction of the nasal spine can be conservative and involve only its lateral surfaces to reduce its width, but it can also involve its length: the spine in some circumstances is a veritable beak which elevates the upper lip (Figs 2.15 and 2.16).

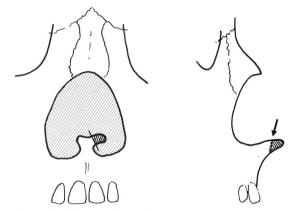

Fig. 2.15 Hypertrophic nasal spine: reduction of projection and width.

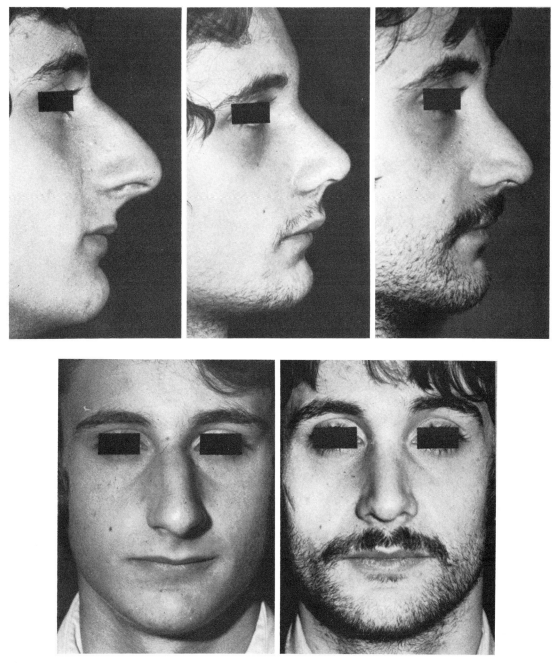

Fig. 2.16 Major naso-labial projection:

— Major projection of the cartilaginous bridge with the effect of suspension over the upper lip which appears too short (left). There is a true rostrum in the area of the nasal spine and a projection of the inferior septum.
— The result at six months (centre top) showing improvement of the lip profile.
— Result at five years (right) with a slight and predictable drop of the nasal tip.

The resection is then carried out with a rongeur, conserving a certain amount of the bone. A total resection of the nasal spine risks causing a retraction of the posterior portion of the columella with a drop of the nasal tip.

The reduction of the nasal spine causes:

— A hollowing of the naso-labial angle and therefore a closure of this angle
— An increase in the height of the upper lip, no longer elevated by the projection of the nasal spine which has been acting like a tent pole.

3. Shortening of the lateral aspects of the nasal spine (Fig. 2.17)

Two cartilaginous obstacles can prevent the elevation of the tip of the nose and the nasal ala: the inferior angles of the triangular cartilages and an excess height of the lateral crura. The reduction of the height of the lateral crura and of the dome can, alone, often provide a slight shortening.

The infero-medial angle of the upper lateral cartilage, which forms a point, is sectioned; but one must be very moderate in this resection, which is carried along a line that is almost horizontal. Fairly often, the lower border of the upper lateral cartilage rolls back on itself, and this can be resected.

As for the reduction in height of the lateral crura, this is carried out at the time of the modification of the cartilages of the nasal tip.

Excess mucosa in this area should not be resected, except, and then with great moderation, in cases of major shortening.

MODELLING OF THE TIP

Modelling of the nasal tip can be done, depending on the preference of the surgeon, either before or after lowering of the cartilaginous bridge.

But it is preferable, particularly in cases where the tip of the nose poses problems (hypertrophy, thick skin, retracted tip), to begin with surgery of the tip, whose new appearance constitutes the structure which determines how much the nasal bridge will be lowered.

The modelling of the alar cartilages plays an essential role in the static state and shape of the tip of the nose; this is one of the important and difficult stages of the operation.

During a rhinoplasty, it is relatively easy to significantly modify the nasal bridge; a very large hump can be resected, and the dorsal nasal skin will usually adapt itself to the new osteocartilaginous framework, because this skin is often thin and elastic. This is not the case at the tip of

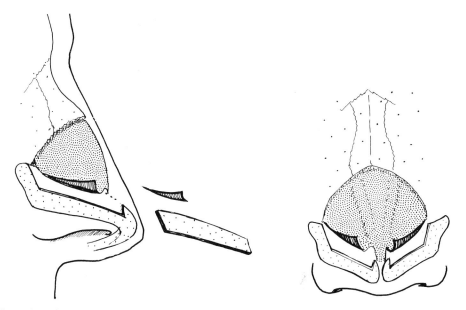

Fig. 2.17   Shortening of the lateral pillars: superior excess of the lateral crus and inferior border of the triangular cartilage.

the nose, where one sees in many cases a difference in thickness: the skin of the tip of the nose is often much thicker than the dorsal nasal skin, and may consequently retract less after the tip cartilages are reduced.

Modifications of the tip of the nose have an effect on the height, width and projection of the tip.

1. Projection

This is determined by the length of the mesial crura; long mesial crura are associated with a long columella, with an accentuated projection of the tip, whereas the converse, short mesial crura, are associated with a short columella with a flat tip (Fig. 2.18).

It is important to estimate from the outset this projection of the tip, which will determine the mode of reduction of the alar cartilages, and particularly to assess its relationship to the nasal bridge.

We should recall that the projection of nasal tip can be reduced by events elsewhere, such as:

— The lowering of the cartilaginous dorsum: a cartilaginous hump with a significant supra-apical projection can act like a 'tent-pole', pushing the tip forward through the skin. One should look out for cases where, after lowering the cartilaginous bridge, the tip of the nose is clearly receding. The phenomenon is further accentuated in cases with thick skin
— resection of the nasal spine
— a backward sliding associated with a interseptocolumellar incision carried down to the nasal spine spine
— reduction in the height of the lateral crura and resection of the tail of the lateral crus, if this is envisaged beforehand.

It is only when this projection is excessive that one has to consider a lowering of the tip by a reduction in height of the mesial crura, that is, *a resection of the domes* which may involve the mesial crura.

2. Width and height

The width and the height of the tip of the nose are related to the height of the lateral crus, the width of the alar dome, and also to the openness of the curve of the cartilaginous dome:

— The cephalic border of the lateral crus determines the height of the tip of the nose.
— The lower border contributes to the maintenance of the nostril opening; it is therefore contraindicated to carry out a total resection of the lateral crus. The reduction of the height of the tip involves resecting the cephalic excess of the lateral crus, leaving a residual height of at least 3–4 mm, which maintains the nostril opening.
— The reduction of the height of the lateral crura in the domes brings about a diminution of the width and a slight rotation of the tip of the nose superiorly.
— The remaining height should be determined according to the 'spring' of the cartilage, and also the thickness of the skin: thin skin retracts much more easily than thick skin and, because of this, requires a more resistant cartilaginous framework.
— The cartilaginous dome provides the form and the width of the lobule (Fig. 2.19):
• an acute dome giving a narrow lobule,
• an obtuse, open dome giving a large and flat lobule.

The desired aim is to obtain a new cartilaginous arch whose modified projection, width and height bring about the desired modification of the tip of the nose.

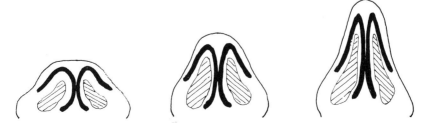

Fig. 2.18 Projection of the nasal tip varies with the height of the mesial crura.

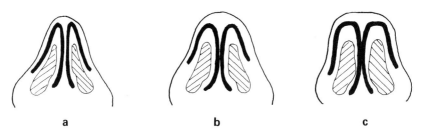

Fig. 2.19 The width of the tip varies with that of the dome. **a.** Acute dome: pinched lobule. **b.** Normal dome. **c.** Wide open dome, wide lobule, square tip.

3. Before determining which techniques to use:

It is useful to examine the tip of the nose to assess its characteristics:

The thickness of the skin, as we have seen, is important.

The 'spring' of the cartilage is assessed by palpation, which makes it possible to differentiate between:

— A tip which is reinforced and well-supported by the alar cartilages; (the alar cartilages are often stronger in men)
— A soft tip, often without firmness, where the cartilaginous support is weak; at operation, one often finds in these cases that the soft cartilages, which dissect poorly and lack firmness, require a cartilage graft for support more often than they do surgery for reduction.

The outer contour, often quite visible, makes it possible to trace on the skin the limits of the lateral crus and the dome, and, sometimes, to note certain singularities of the lateral crura (see section on Anatomy).

One also notes the appearance of the alar crease and the presence or absence of a marked depression along the ala; such a depression constitutes a contraindication to resection of the tail of the lateral crus which serves only to accentuation this depression.

The lower limit of the lateral crus can be assessed by an intra-nasal examination, and one may be surprised by the differences between one case and the next (see section on anatomy of the alar cartilages). This lower limit is important, because it is the site of a marginal or infracartilaginous incision if this is envisaged. *The lower limit of the lateral crus does not follow the nostril border* (Figs 2.20 and 2.21).

The length of the columella, and the projection of the tip are also noted.

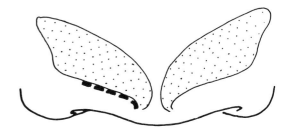

Fig. 2.20 The inferior border of the lateral crus does not follow the nostril border from which it remains at a distance.

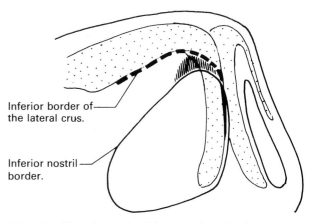

Inferior border of the lateral crus.

Inferior nostril border.

Fig. 2.21 The soft triangle of Converse (cross hatched zone), which should be preserved during the marginal incision.

THE DIRECT APPROACH

The direct approach exposes the domes to direct view, thanks to a 'bucket handle' exteriorisation. This has the advantages of enabling us:

1. To see the shape of the domes, to locate the line of the summit and to identify certain singularities.
2. To appreciate the differences between the two sides and to judge the degree of asymmetry.
3. To measure and carry out exactly the resection required, leaving symmetrical cartilages: the important thing is what remains behind!
4. To equilibrate the domes as one sees them and as one feels them.
5. To see, in cases of section of the dome, the anterior extremities of the mesial and lateral crura; one can then round-off the angles, and prevent a residual anterior Polly-beak deformity.

The direct approach is indicated:

— In difficult cases and, particularly, in secondary rhinoplasties.
— In asymmetries where the exposure of the cartilages makes it possible to carry out a resection which leaves the cartilages in a symmetrical state.
— When the cartilaginous surface is irregular, with protuberances and depressions.
— In cases where a modification of the shape of the dome is indicated.

The marginal incision (Fig. 2.22) should be very precisely made, with the incision line following the inferior border of the lateral crus and of the dome. The incision is perpendicular to the skin, and the scalpel blade seeks contact with the cartilage. At the level of the dome, the incision is 2–3 mm from the nostril border, leaving free a small cutaneous zone free of cartilage which constitutes the border of the anterior sill of the vestibule.

At the level of the columella, the incision is 1 mm from the nostril border which it extends along for about 5 mm. It continues laterally and passes medially following the inferior border of the lateral crus.

The dissection is then carried out with sharp or blunt fine-pointed scissors; it frees the superficial surface of the cartilages from the skin covering, which makes it possible to exteriorise the cartilage as a 'bucket handle'.

The exteriorisation (Fig. 2.23). A double hook stabilises the nostril border, and a single hook pulls the inferior border of the dome downwards, permitting the exteriorisation of the cartilage lined by the vestibular skin. An instrument (end of the scissor or the handle of the hook) is placed inside this 'bucket handle' loop to maintain the exteriorisation; the same manoeuvre is carried out on the opposite side.

The two cartilages are thus exposed almost completely. In fact, the superior portion and, particularly, the supero-lateral portion of the lateral crura are less well exposed, and it is sometimes preferable to approach them initially in a retrograde fashion.

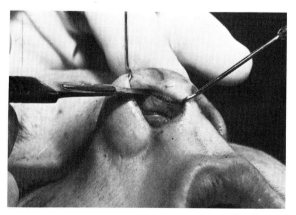
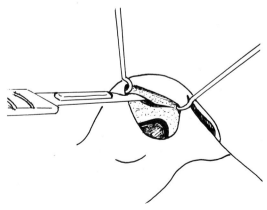

Fig. 2.22 Marginal incision.

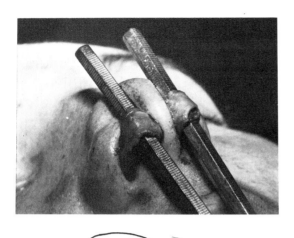

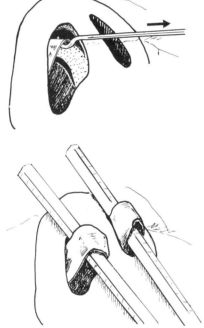

Fig. 2.23 Exteriorisation of the alar cartilages.

After excision of the fragments of fatty tissue which cover them, the cartilages have a pearly-white, smooth and shiny appearance, and, if the undermining between the domes and the adjacent mesial crura has been carried out symmetrically, can be seen and studied simultaneously and the two sides compared.

The modifications of the domes and the lateral crura are then carried out under direct vision, with measurements made with a small caliper. Measurements are made of the area to be resected but also, particularly, of the height of the

cartilage to remain behind, which should be the same on both sides.

In the case of resection of the domes, the ends of the cartilage at the level of the section are rounded off.

This method is excellent and very often used; however:

— The incision does not permit the smallest error in its location which should follow the inferior border of the alar cartilage

— The exteriorised 'bucket handle' should be perfectly repositioned and held in place either by catgut sutures or by packing to prevent any separation of the wound edges; swelling can be more pronounced along the upper border of the incision and can be responsible for this separation.

THE RETROGRADE METHOD

The retrograde method aims to avoid marginal incision by everting the lateral crus and the dome after an undermining between skin and cartilage (Fig. 2.24).

A double hook is placed along the nostril border, and counterpressure is exerted by the middle finger; the undermining is then carried out with a blunt, curved-tipped scissors;

— The undermining of the lateral crus is carried out down to the inferior border of the cartilage

— The undermining of the dome is carried out through the opposite nostril.

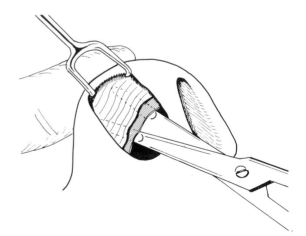

Fig. 2.24 Retrograde undermining of the lateral crus, carried out through the ipsilateral nostril.

The area of undermining. This is carried out flush with the cartilage in the case of a thin nose with thin skin, and near the skin if the nose is thick.

The extent of the undermining (Fig. 2.25):

— Inferiorly, this reaches the inferior border of the lateral crus and the dome

— Laterally, it is extended according to how much one wants to resect of the tail of the lateral crus; in fact, we are not in favour of this resection because it risks creating a zone of weakness where the spring of the cartilaginous attachment is useful

— In rare cases, where the ala appears high and without form, and the alar crease disappears due to excessive alar cartilage, the resection can involve the tail of the lateral crus

— Medially, the domes are separated and the undermining is carried out as far as the first few millimetres of the mesial crus.

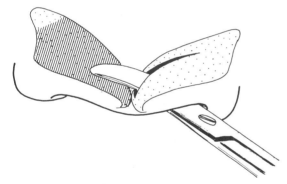

Fig. 2.25 Retrograde undermining carried out through the contralateral nostril.

An undermining correctly carried out facilitates the eversion of the cartilage.

Eversion of the cartilage. A single hook is placed at each end of the lateral crus, and the latter is turned outwards on its hinge (the inferior border of the lateral crus).

Two choices are possible:

1. Conservation of the continuity of the dome.
2. Section/resection of the dome.

In the first case (Fig. 2.26). The dissection is performed on the lateral crus by using sharp pointed scissors, separating the vestibular skin from the cartilage to enable resection of the superior excess of the lateral crus.

The plane of dissection may be:

— Subperichondrial if the cartilage is sufficiently rigid, or

— Supraperichondrial, that is, leaving the perichondreum adherent to the cartilage which is thus more resistant and can be worked on better; but in this situation the undermining is more difficult, and a tear in the vestibular skin is possible.

The approach by 'simple eversion', without section of the domes, is an elegant and conservative method.

The modifications are, however, limited for us to cases where one wants to obtain a slight and subtle modification of the tip, aiming to 'model' it by reducing the projection very slightly or not at all.

In the second case. Section of the domes is carried out (Fig. 2.27a).

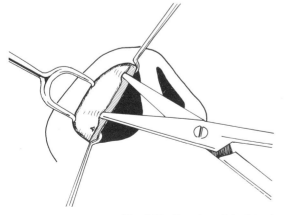

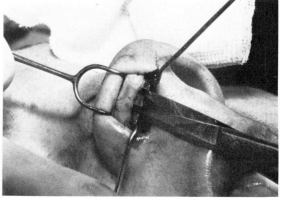

Fig. 2.26 Eversion of the lateral crus and undermining of the vestibular skin.

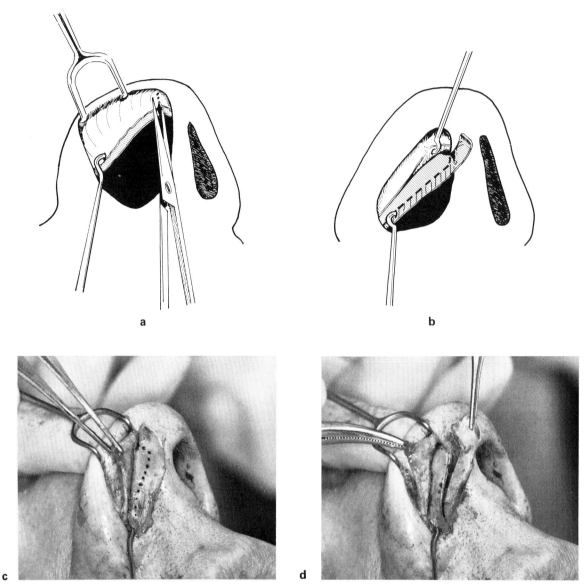

Fig. 2.27   Section of the domes. **a.** Simultaneous section of the cartilage and the vestibular skin. **b.** and **c.** Exteriorisation of the lateral crus and the dome. **d.** 'Hockey stick' resection of the superior excess of the lateral crus.

This section is carried out on the vestibular skin and the cartilage, which are sectioned simultaneously, as far as the inferior border of the cartilage, i.e., 2–3 mm from the nostril rim.

The section is carried out medial to the dome, encroaching on the medial crus to a degree dependent on the extent of the desired lowering.

This section makes possible a complete and perfect eversion (Fig. 2.27b,c,d) of the lateral crus and of the dome, so that one can then carry out a

resection of the superior excess of the lateral crus and a resection of the dome; the resected fragment has the shape of a hockey stick. The ends of the lateral crus and of the mesial crus are rounded-off in order to avoid a noticeable projection under the skin.

This is a delicate procedure, in which an excessive ablation of the dome should be avoided; it can lead to a pinched tip when the external section is carried out too far laterally. The freed cartilages should be replaced with care, and sutures placed with precision.

THE LOW INTRACARTILAGINOUS INCISION (Millard-Peck)

The advantage of this technique is its rapidity, since:

— It involves a low, intracartilaginous incision 3 mm from the lower border of the lateral crus
— It does not require retrograde undermining.

It is useful when the skin has little suppleness, and the nostril orifices are small. But one must take care to locate properly the lower border of the lateral crus in order to avoid an excessive resection of it. In general, it is preferable to leave a greater height to the lateral crus if the cartilage lacks tonicity and spring, if there is already a tendency to collapse (narrow nostril orifices, a lateral crus concave on its outer surface), and if the projection of the tip is insufficient.

A PROCEDURE: EXPOSURE OF THE DOME WITH A 'BUCKET HANDLE' FLAP THROUGH A CONTRALATERAL APPROACH (Aiach)

It is possible, in certain cases, to exteriorise the dome and the adjacent portion of the lateral crus through the opposite nostril. When the reduction of the alar cartilages is carried out by a retrograde approach, it is useful, at the end of this stage, to check the remaining height of the domes by placing a double hook at the summit of the op-

posite nostril and then exerting a digital counterpressure on the dome towards this nostril. The exposure is sometimes so good as to lead us in a number of cases to carry out the modifications of the alar cartilages through this approach; this requires that the skin be supple, and the nostrils of a normal size. The advantages of this technique is that it permits exposure of the dome and a portion of the lateral crus to direct view, without a marginal incision.

1. The stage of the tip

This is normally begun by a retrograde undermining extending as far as the lower border of the lateral crura, at the level of the domes and between the medial crura in their upper half; this permits a correct mobilisation of the cartilaginous domes — both in relation to one other and in relation to the cutaneous layers (Fig. 2.25).

2. The next stage

This consists of:

a. A subperichondrial undermining (carried out with sharp-pointed scissors) extending as far as possible towards the dome without exerting excessive force (Fig. 2.26);

b. Resection of a cartilaginous strip from the superior border of the lateral crus. This resection is done from lateral to medial; the strip of cartilage can be resected immediately or left in place provisionally, attached to the dome (Fig. 2.28) (which permits one to better understand the procedure).

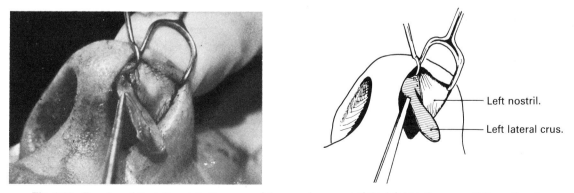

Left nostril.

Left lateral crus.

Fig. 2.28 Eversion of the left nostril. Exposure of the superior excess of the left lateral crus, partially sectioned.

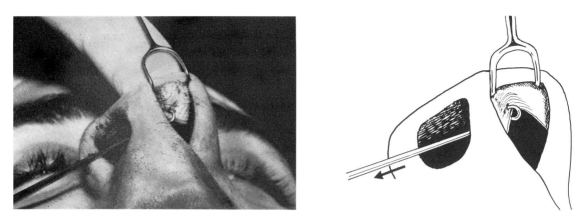

Fig. 2.29 The skin hook is placed in the vestibular skin of the left dome.

The height of the lateral crus can be verified and completed later.

3. Exposure of the dome

This can now be carried out (for purposes of description we will describe the exposure of the left dome through the right nostril, (Fig. 2.29).

1. A double hook is placed at the summit of the left nostril orifice.

2. A single hook is introduced into the intersepto-columellar space, and grasps the free border of the vestibular skin facing the left dome.

3. Then, aided by pressure from the middle finger, this hook pulls the left dome into the right nostril which will be accompanied by the beginning of an invagination of the skin in the region of the left dome towards the right nostril (Fig. 2.30).

4. In this way, the dome passes in a horizontal plane through a rotation of 180° around the axis of the columella, and enters the concavity of the right alar arch.

5. The outer surface of the cartilage is then cleared of the fatty tissue of varying thickness which covers it, in order to obtain a cartilaginous surface which is clean and smooth and whose borders can be easily seen (Fig. 2.31).

6. One can then easily note:

— The dome whose position is *inverted* (the superior border lies below). However, the trick of leaving the superior strip of the lateral crus in place makes it possible to recognise, after the rotation, that this strip corresponds to the superior excess of the lateral crus, now located inferiorly.

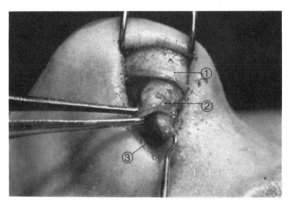

Fig. 2.30 Under the vestibular skin of the right dome (1), the left dome appears (2), pulled by a single hook in the right nostril (3). The hook pulls on the vestibular skin separated from the cartilaginous dome by undermining with sharp pointed scissors.

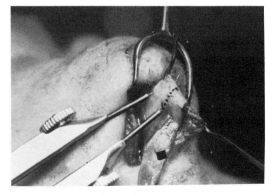

Fig. 2.31 Exposure of the left dome in the right nostril. The upper hook holds the lower border of the left dome; the lower hook is in the vestibular skin next to the superior border of the left dome; the superior excess of the left lateral crus, which has been partially sectioned is seen inferiorly (black square); measurement of the height of the remaining cartilage.

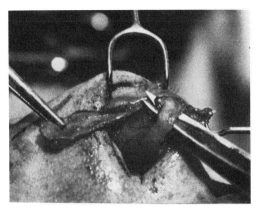

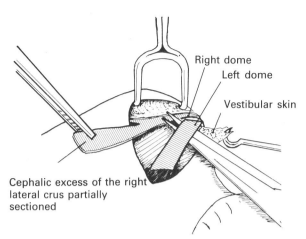

Right dome
Left dome

Vestibular skin

Cephalic excess of the right
lateral crus partially
sectioned

Fig. 2.32 Exposure of the left cartilaginous dome (contralateral 'bucket handle'). The dome appears under the tip of the scissors. The right dome passes as a bridge above the left dome.

— One can note equally well:
- the lower third of the mesial crus
- the anterior portion of the lateral crus whose retracted medial edge indicates the position of the dome.

After the dissection of the dome, a 'bucket handle' can be made (Fig. 2.32), and the resections and modifications which are required can then be carried out under direct view with measurements being taken of the remaining cartilage:

— Either by diminution of the height of the cartilaginous dome extending along the lateral crus
— Or by multiple vertical incisions, parallel or staggered (without undermining the vestibular skin).

This procedure, which avoids the the marginal incision, enables a reduction of the height of the lateral crura and the domes with direct measurement of the height of the remaining cartilage. It also permits one to carry out weakening incisions of the domes (either parallel or staggered incisions).

The ideal indication is provided by a case of moderate hypertrophy of the tip of the nose (Fig. 2.33).

What to do with the nasal tip?

The shape of the nasal tip is determined by the shape of the alar cartilages themselves which have a varying amount of spring, and which are covered by skin of variable thickness; it is essentially in the modifications carried out on these cartilages that the problem lies.

Surgery of the nasal tip constitutes the first operative stage, and the modifications to be performed on the nasal bridge (lowering of the profile line, reduction in width) should be kept in mind in order to harmonise them with the width and projection of the nasal tip. The surgeon should be equally aware of all manoeuvres which involve a lowering the nasal tip.

The indications may be summarised thus:

a. Excessive projection. A retrograde or direct approach permitting:

— The resection of the domes with a variable resection of the mesial crus
— The reduction of the height of the lateral crura (Fig. 2.34).

b. Increased projection but without excess. The reduction of the height of the domes and of the lateral crura may be sufficient, particularly if one approaches the rhinoplasty conservatively (Fig. 2.35).

The low intracartilaginous incision may be indicated, since resection of the excess lateral crus is sufficient to slightly lower the tip.

c. Projection appears normal (Fig. 2.36).
There is a risk of diminution of the projection of the nasal tip, and this is greater when the columella is short or the cartilaginous bridge is

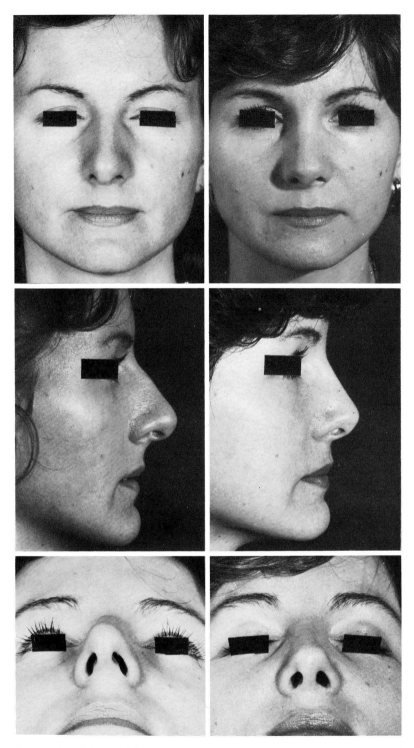

Fig. 2.33 Moderate hypertrophy of the tip of the nose.

— Tip: reduction of the superior excess of the lateral crura (without section of the domes) by a contralateral approach.
— Reduction of the osteocartilaginous bridge (osteotome).
— Lateral osteotomy in an 'ascending curve'.
— Insertion over the bridge of a fragment of crushed septal cartilage.

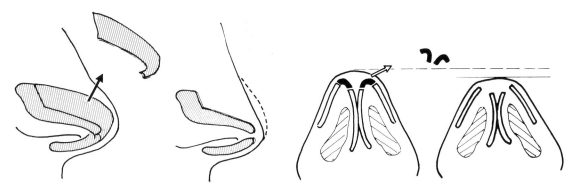

Fig. 2.34 Excessive projection: the resection in continuity of the superior excess of the lateral crus and of the dome permits the removal of a 'hockey-stick' shaped cartilaginous fragment.

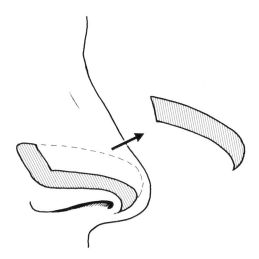

Fig. 2.35 Projection is slightly increased: the height of the dome is reduced.

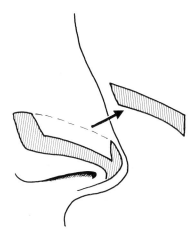

Fig. 2.36 Normal projection: the height of the dome is conserved.

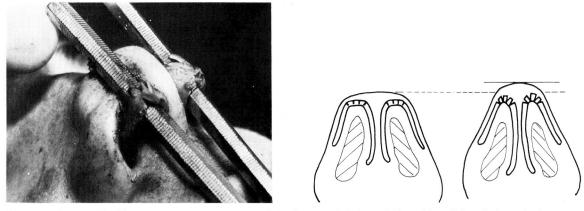

Fig. 2.37 Staggered incision permitting the weakening of the domes and their modelling with a slight gain in projection.

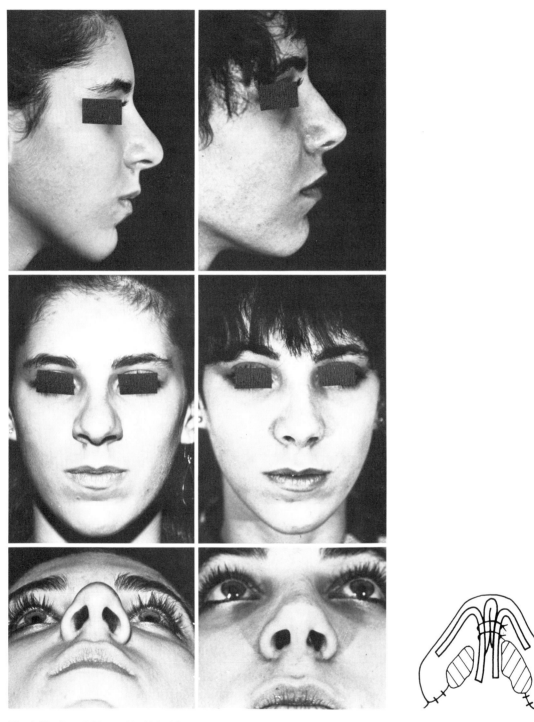

Fig. 2.37 (cont.) Nose with thick skin, globular tip:

— Extramucosal dissection.
— *Tip*: exteriorisation of the domes; reduction of the superior excess of the lateral crura, and staggered cartilaginous incisions in the domes; lowering of the cartilaginous bridge.
— Median and lateral osteotomy in an 'ascending curve'.
— Cartilage graft to the tip: a fragment of the lateral crus is folded over upon itself and placed between the two mesial crura to reinforce the projection of the tip of the nose.
— *Alae*: cutaneous resection, 3 mm in width.

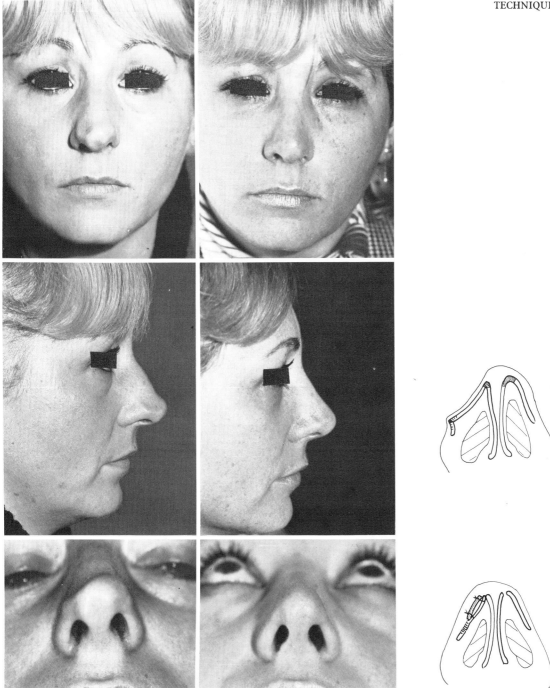

Fig. 2.38 Projecting and asymmetrical tip.

— Marginal incision and exposure of the domes and the lateral crura.
— Re-establishment of symmetry by a graft of a fragment of the lateral crus sutured to the right lateral crus. Asymmetrical resection of the domes.
— Reduction of a projection to the left by cartilaginous incisions.
— Reduction of the hump; shortening; lateral osteotomies.
— Cartilage graft over the bridge.

itself prominent; the reduction of the height should be performed on the lateral crura and not on the domes. A supporting cartilage graft is at times useful at the end of the operation.

d. Projection is insufficient. The use of cartilage grafts is preferable to procedures which involve sectioning the domes laterally and suturing them in the midline.

e. A wide bulbous tip (Fig. 5.25).

If the projection is normal, one can:

— To a limited extent, confine oneself to a reduction of the height of the lateral crura and the domes without sectioning them, which weakens them just enough to model the tip.
— Sometimes, it will be necessary to weaken the domes by using vertical incisions, parallel or staggered, involving only the cartilage (Fig. 2.37).

Finally, in certain cases, the excessive projection requires a resection of the domes, this time by resection from the mesial crura (Fig. 2.34).

f. Asymmetry or anomalies of the tip. A direct approach with exteriorisation of the cartilages is the only method that permits a correction of the defects by resection or grafts (Fig. 2.38).

g. Very pointed domes. In cases of a very pointed dome, with a projecting and sometimes pinched tip, it can be sufficient to resect the projecting portion of the dome or to crush it by using flat-jawed forceps (Fig. 2.39). It is sometimes necessary to place a graft on top of the domes to widen the tip of the nose.

The role of the skin is very important

— A thin skin makes the slightest projection or irregularity of the cartilages apparent, which is an

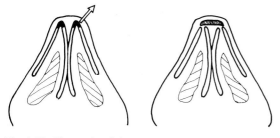

Fig. 2.39 Very pointed domes: correction by discreet resection with or without cartilage grafts.

indication for conserving at least 4–5 mm of the height of the lateral crus.
— A thick, heavy skin can, by dint of its weight play a role in the diminution of the projection of the nasal tip; one determines by the spring of the cartilage how much to reduce the height of the remaining cartilage (up to 3 mm).

However, one should always be prudent, because thick skin adapts itself less well over the cartilaginous framework in spite of defatting carried out on the deep surface of the skin intended to remove the sometimes numerous fatty globules.

RESECTION OF THE OSTEOCARTILAGINOUS HUMP AND REDUCTION OF THE NASAL BRIDGE

DETERMINATION OF THE AMOUNT TO RESECT

This data is the most important and the most difficult to determine; it is this which enables us to obtain the desired result. The 'skin' factor is of course of considerable importance.

The reduction of the nasal bridge depends on several factors which are analysed during the initial examination:

— The projection of the bridge and the length of the nose
— The width of the bridge
— The desires of the patient.

1. The projection of the nasal bridge

This should always be assessed keeping in mind its width. In general, one can carry out a greater reduction when the bridge is narrow and the nose fine. The problem is not the same for noses with a wide bridge, where the reduction will be moderate.

The nasal profile can be studied on a lateral photograph or xeroradiogram at different levels:

— Naso-frontal angle
— High point of the nasal hump
— Supratip region
— Nasal tip.

• At the level of the naso-frontal angle, deepen-

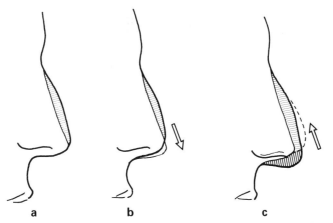

Fig. 2.40 **a.** Nose of normal length. **b.** Short nose: resection of the hump and slight lengthening. **c.** Long nose: Shortening and resection of the hump.

ing is indicated if the glabella is flat with straight forehead-nose profile. However, the reduction of the osseous bridge (the hump and the osseous root) should take into account an element which is often neglected: The projection of the eyeballs; if this is marked, the reduction of the bridge should be less.

We will comment here on an element which has a completely different effect! In certain cases of naso-maxillary hollowing, there is the effect of hypertelorism. The eyes appear overly separated and a bone graft reduces this effect by giving height to the nasal bridge.

● At the level of the high point of the nasal hump: it is here that the length of the bridge is important. Three different situations can occur (Fig. 2.40):

1. The nose is of normal length. No shortening is necessary and resection of the osteocartilaginous hump can be carried out according to the plan established on photographs or X-rays.

2. The nose is short. It is desirable to lengthen it slightly, but in this case, the reduction of the bridge is limited to obtaining a straight bridge; excessive resection involves an elevation of the tip of the nose. One can see this phenomenon during the insertion of a cartilage graft along the nasal bridge, where the impression of lengthening is created by a rotation of the tip inferiorly and by an upward displacement of the naso-frontal indentation.

3. The nose is too long, with a falling tip, and, according to the preoperative study, it should be considerably shortened. In this particular case, one shortens the nose before carrying out the reduction of the bridge which can then be better evaluated.

In fact, the elevation of the tip of the nose involves a partial effacement of the hump and can result in a saddle deformity if the hump is initially excessively resected.

2. The factor of the skin

This is particularly important in the last case above. Age, and the thickness and elasticity of the skin should be carefully considered before any nasal reduction. During a reduction of the bridge, cutaneous retraction permits the skin and soft tissues to adapt themselves to the new osteo-cartilaginous framework; it is important therefore that, as during an advancement, one carries out enough undermining to permit the skin to slide over the underlying osteocartilaginous plane.

The greater the reduction of the profile and the greater the shortening, the more extensive should be the undermining.

In the case of a thick, seborrhoeic skin, the retraction may not be as satisfactory, with the possibility of a Polly-beak deformity, and it may be preferable here to carry out a moderate reduction of the profile, followed by a reimplantation of the tailored hump.

The reduction of the nasal bridge should, in any case, take into account the limits of the reduction of the nasal tip.

3. The 'desire' of the patient

This is a factor which should be kept in mind, but considered together with all the other data, particularly if the patient wants a major modification. These cases need to be treated moderately and one should explain to the patient the reasons why the surgeon may need to carry out less of a reduction than the patient desires.

RESECTION OF THE OSTEOCARTILAGINOUS HUMP

This should always be carried out to a slightly lesser extent than the planned resection; it may then easily be finished with serrated scissors in the cartilaginous portion and with the rasp on the osseous portion in order to obtain the desired result.

The resection of the osteocartilaginous hump involves two stages:

1. Section of the cartilages
2. Section of the bone.

1. Cartilaginous sections

a. Section of the upper lateral cartilages (Fig. 2.41):

— An Aufricht retractor is introduced into the right nostril (if one is right-handed) and kept strictly in the midline, retracting the skin. The section of the upper lateral cartilages is then carried out under direct view with serrated scissors or scalpel.

— The lower blade of the serrated scissors is introduced between the mucosal dome, which it pushes slightly backwards, and the under surface of the cartilaginous septo-triangular junction. The upper blade of the scissors is positioned between the skin and the cartilage, and the scissors, having made contact with, and thereby located, the deep portion of the cartilaginous junction, are oriented horizontally. The section is made with a simple snip of the scissors, pushing with the scissors as far as the inferior border of the nasal bone which one should feel through the instrument.

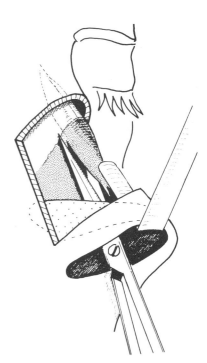

Fig. 2.41 Section of the upper lateral cartilages with serrated scissors.

— A symmetrical procedure is carried out on the opposite side.

— The quantity of triangular cartilage resected initially is always somewhat less than that which one has foreseen.

b. Section of the anterior septal border. This is carried out in the same fashion, and the line of the section should be situated along the same plane as the preceding sections (Fig. 2.42).

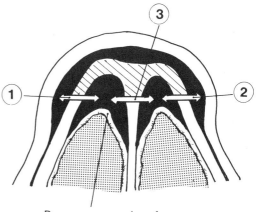

Dome or mucosal roof

Fig. 2.42 Cartilaginous sections: ① and ② upper lateral cartilages; ③ septum.

2. Resection of the bone

This completes the resection of the osteocartilaginous hump. The difficulties encountered in the precise resection of the nasal bony hump, particularly at the level of the naso-frontal angle, stem partly from the deep location of the latter, but also from the density of the bone at this level.

What to use? Rasp or osteotome?

a. Rasp

Use of the rasp is indicated if one wants to lower a small hump (Figs 2.43 and 5.12):

— There is certainly no risk of excessive resection, but on the one hand, the naso-frontal angle is difficult to hollow out, and on the other hand, one needs to be very careful in the choice of this instrument and its use in order to avoid tears and disinsertions of the upper lateral cartilages in their upper portion.

— Thus, the rasp should be used in an oblique direction, which is less traumatic for the upper lateral cartilages.

— Certain rasps work only from below upwards and are also less traumatic.

When a rasp is used, the reduction of the cartilaginous bridge (septum-triangular cartilage) is done secondarily, after the reduction of the bony bridge.

b. Osteotome

Use of the osteotome permits:

— A monobloc resection of the osteocartilaginous hump, which is often very useful if a reinsertion is envisaged (a tailored hump, or a hump with its longitudinal fragments removed). The resection of more hump than was anticipated is less of a problem in consequence.

— To obtain clean osseous section lines without the multiple small bits of debris caused by the rasp.

— To be able to easily deepen the naso-frontal angle when this is indicated.

The use of the osteotome with an exterior guide-shank permits a greater precision in the desired

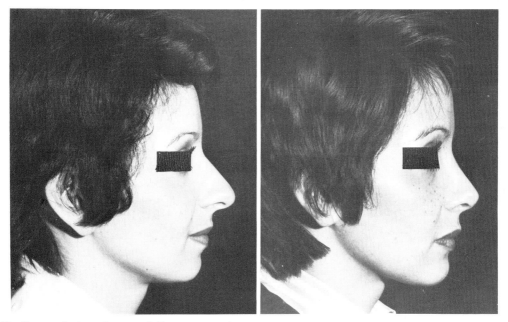

Fig. 2.43 Osteocartilaginous hump and discrete retrogenia.

— Discrete retrogenia: endobuccal approach and placement of a silicon prosthesis.
— Nose: rectangular shortening increasing anteriorly (3 mm); reduction of the nasal spine. Tip: reduction of the lateral crura and triangular resection of the lower border of the mesial crura. Rasping over the bony bridge; reduction of the cartilaginous bridge with serrated scissors.

resection of bone, particularly at the naso-frontal angle.

c. Drawbacks of bony resection by the osteotome are:

— On the one hand, the possibility of fracturing or shattering the nasal bones — this can be avoided by having an osteotome which has been perfectly sharpened
— On the other hand, this method may be more difficult for a beginner. The technique demands a great deal of precision, with the instrument being guided by direct view (in its direction) and by palpation of the lateral edges of the blade of the osteotome.

d. Analysis of the lateral X-ray and the use of the shank-guided osteotome (Fig. 2.44).

The analysis of the lateral nasal X-ray when the nasal bridge is straight shows that the osteocartilaginous profile is slightly convex, and also that the thickness of the soft tissues at the level of the nasion is variable (3.5–9.5 mm).

If, at the point of impaction of the osteotome at the lower border of the nasal bones, one can properly establish the depth of the instrument by palpation of its edges, this is not the case as one approaches the nasion; here, the thickness of the soft tissues (about 7.5 mm on average) is noticeably increased by the anaesthetic infiltration, and, in addition, the retractor or osteotome displaces the landmarks and the cutaneous marks which had previously been made, rendering them imprecise. This is why a landmark at this level should not be cutaneous but bony, and this can be made extremely simply and precisely by using a straight needle fixed horizontally through the root of the nose, and passing just over the nasal bone at a point very close to the nasion (Fig. 2.45a). This is the first important point, the second being to direct the osteotome towards this fixed landmark, or a little behind it if one wants to deepen the naso-frontal angle, using an exterior shank guide. The osteotome with the shank guide which we recommend is a straight, T-shaped osteotome with an average width of about 16 mm; this is adequate for the great majority of nasal bony humps (Fig. 2.44). The outer edges of the blade are smooth, which avoids the possibility of damaging the undersurface of the skin.

The midportion of the instrument on one side has an enlargement which has two uses:

— On the one hand, it makes possible a better grip on instrument, in the place where it is usually held
— On the other hand, it permits the passage of an exterior shank-guide which also passes through the adjacent lateral branch of the 'T'. *This shank-guide can slide while remaining in the plane of the osteotome.*

Its lower portion (near the cutting end of the osteotome), is pointed, but blunt and located 7–8 mm from the lateral edge of the osteotome, which corresponds to a distance greater than the thickness of the soft tissues in the region of the lateral portions of the nose.

The upper end (above the horizontal bar) is curved off at a right angle. The curved portion is always facing laterally for two reasons:

— Firstly, it permits the assistant to tap with a mallet;
— Secondly, to be sure that the guide, which is semi-rigid, has its lower end in the plane of the osteotome.

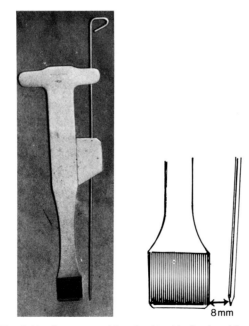

8mm

Fig. 2.44 Osteotome with a shank-guide developed by G. Aiach (made by Micro-France), (width of 12–16 mm).

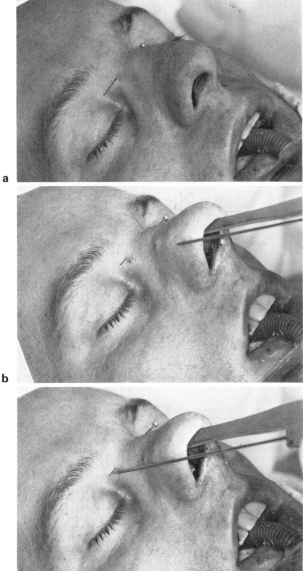

a

b

c

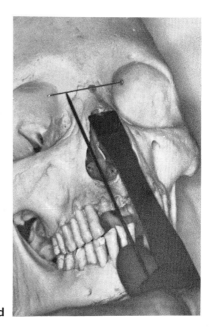

d

Fig. 2.45 Resection of the osseous hump using an osteotome with a shank-guide. **a.** Precise localisation of the bony nasion. **b.** The shank being retracted, the osteotome is placed at the inferior edge of the nasal bones. **c.** and **d.** The end of the guide goes back to the level of the nasion, providing an adequate orientation for the osteotome.

Before use. The precision of the instrument should be checked; for this, the lower end of the shank, which is pointed but blunt, is passed beyond the cutting end and one checks to see that it is located along the prolongation of the latter. The shank is then drawn back several centimetres and the resection of the nasal hump can be carried out.

Technique. With the shank retracted 4–5 cm, the osteotome is placed against the inferior portion of the nasal bone. The position of the osteotome against the inferior border of the nasal bone can be checked easily by the operator's other hand through the very thin skin at this level (Fig. 2.45b).

The sliding shank is then progressively advanced until it makes contact with the needle previously placed at the root of the nose, which indicates by its horizontality the bony level of the nasion (N); this makes it possible to orientate the osteotome in a precise fashion towards point N (Fig. 2.45c and d).

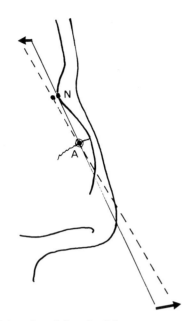

Fig. 2.46 Orientation of the axis of the osteotome according to the osseous resection desired.

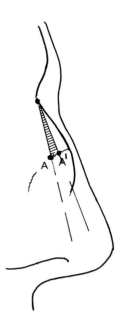

Fig. 2.47 Point of impact of the osteotome at the lower border of the nasal bones. The bony excess to be rasped away is represented by the cross hatched zone, when the osteotome is impacted too superficially (A_1).

If the osseous resection is to be carried out to point N, which is most often the case, the direction of the osteotome is maintained, and the shank is progressively retracted as one carries out the resection.

If the osseous resection needs to be greater at the level of the naso-frontal angle, which is rare, the osteotome is slightly elevated, and pivoted at the level of its point of impaction, A, in such a way that the distance between the lower end of the shank and the needle corresponds to the thickness of the desired in resection at this level (Fig. 2.46).

This technique enables greater precision, but one must be aware of certain factors which are causes of imprecision.

First of all, there is the reference point N. The needle should be sufficiently rigid (a diameter of 0.7 mm is suitable), and should be strictly horizontal, flush with the bone.

As concerns the level of attack of the osteotome to the lower border of the nasal bone (Fig. 2.47):

— It is sometimes correct to have point A the point of attack of the osteotome to the lower border of the nasal bone.
— If this level is a bit superficial (point A^1) the rasp can easily complete the necessary resection which is carried out essentially on the lower portions of the nasal bones, which at this level are thinner and therefore easier to rasp.

— Finally, if this level is deeper, a graft of cartilage or retailored hump can be considered, which underlines the importance of resecting the hump in one piece.

In summary

The resection of the bony hump can be carried out:

1. *With a rasp* if it is minimal.
2. *With a straight osteotome* for the usual type of hump. Use of the shank-guide is particularly indicated in large humps because it can guide the resection to the exact point desired.

The resection should be slightly less than that which had been planned:

1. At the level of the triangular and septal cartilages, where adjustment can be made with the scissors or with the scalpel.
2. At the level of the bone, where it can be carried out easily with the rasp.

EXAMINATION OF THE OSTEOCARTILAGINOUS HUMP

This is an important stage which provides considerable information (Fig. 2.48).

The deep surface of the hump permits one to verify:

• Whether the extramucosal dissection has been correctly carried out; there should be no vestige of mucus in the lateral-septal grooves
• Whether the hump has been resected in a symmetrical fashion.

— The midline corresponds to the septum (assuming a straight nose without septal deviation)
— The lines of the cuts are symmetrical and clean
— At the level of the upper lateral cartilages, one can also verify the symmetry of the resection.

On the superficial surface, one can note the presence of soft tissue debris.

The hump is placed in a cup containing saline solution. It may be used for reinsertion at the end of the operation; otherwise, it can be kept in a sterile tube under refrigeration for three weeks to a month (after carefully 'stripping' the hump on both surfaces).

Conclusions from the examination of the nasal hump:

• The resection has been symmetrical: no further resection is necessary but it may be useful to perform further, with minimal resections in order to arrive at the desired profile:

— At the level of the upper lateral cartilages, one can proceeed with resections of minimal symmetrical fragments.

— At the level of the bone, the rasp, used obliquely to avoid disinserting or traumatising the upper lateral cartilages, makes it possible to carry out the necessary adjustment. This adjustment is easy in the inferior portion of the nasal bone, where the bone is thin, and easy to rasp; on the other hand, it becomes more difficult at the level of the naso-frontal angle where the bone is much more thick and dense. When further resection is necessary at this level, it is often simpler and more reliable to carry it out using a chisel with a short bevel (MacIndoe or Neivert).

• The resection has been asymmetrical: the symmetry will be obtained at the level of the upper lateral cartilages, where it is carried out under direct vision, as well as at the level of the bone where it is controlled by palpation.

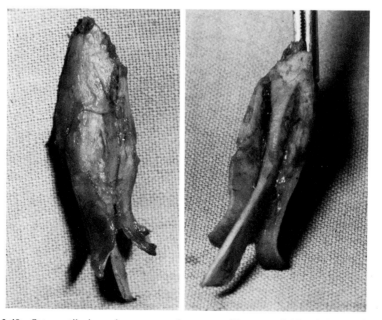

Fig. 2.48 Osteocartilaginous hump resected as a monobloc: superficial and deep surfaces.

● There are mucosal fragments adherent to the hump.

This is not bothersome if a reinsertion of the hump is not planned. Indeed, until recently, many surgeons carried out a deliberate section of the hump at the same time as that of the mucosa, often with good results.

What should one do in a case of excessive resection of the osteocartilaginous hump? It is sufficient to retailor, that is, to reduce the resected hump (after having removed the soft tissue from both surfaces) and to reinsert it.

OSTEOTOMY

After resection of the osteocartilaginous hump, the nose appears wider, and the bridge has a flat plateau. The aim of the osteotomies is to bring together the two bony segments in order to obtain a harmonious bridge which is neither too wide, nor too pinched, and which is regular, without disturbing of the supra-orbital lines. The bringing together of the nasal bones by osteotomies is therefore an important manoeuvre in the reconstitution of the bony roof. Because bleeding can be considerable, it is preferable to carry this out at the end of the operation.

The osteotomy can be done in three stages (Fig. 2.49):

— *First stage:* medial or sagittal osteotomy which creates a zone of weakness in the area where one wants to make the high fracture.
— *Second stage:* lateral or posterior osteotomy carried out at the level of the nasal process of the maxilla; we will see the variations on this.
— *Third stage:* a superior osteotomy or high fracture carried out by medial luxation of the bony segment. The precision of the high fracture depends on that of the two preceding stages.

It is after these osteotomies have been done that one individualises the *osteocartilaginous flap* which is mobilised and shifted medially (see Anatomy section). The mobility of this flap varies from one case to another, and can result in an insufficient or excessive displacement.

From a horizontal section, passing through the mid portion of the nasal bone, one can see (Fig. 2.50):

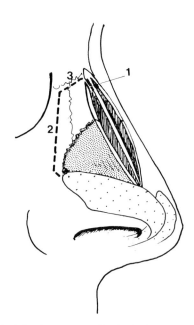

Fig. 2.49 The three stages of a classical osteotomy: 1. median osteotomy; 2. lateral osteotomy; 3. high fracture.

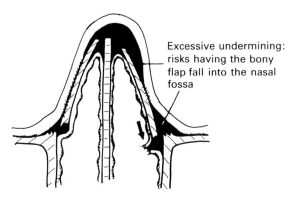

Excessive undermining: risks having the bony flap fall into the nasal fossa

Fig. 2.50 Horizontal section at the level of the nasal bones.

— On the one hand, that the nasal bones do not rest on a platform
— On the other hand, that after the osteotomies, the edge of the maxilla along the osteotomy line may be too thin to be able to maintain the bony flap, which tends to recoil slightly, and sometimes to fall into the nasal fossa.

It is obviously the high osseous portion of the osteocartilaginous flap which provides greater stability to the latter. An excessive subperiosteal undermining at the level of the bony flap can result in a recoil, or in certain cases, even a fall

Table 2.1 Factors influencing the stabling of the bony flap

	Factors leading to instability of the bony flap	Factors leading to stability of the bony flap
Anatomical factors	Short nasal bones (there is a risk of the bony flap falling into the nasal fossae with a cartilaginous pinching)	Long nasal bones Thick nasal process of maxilla
Specific factors	Wide nose, wide nasal fossae Bone bulging laterally (because the displacement is more extensive)	Narrow nose, or one of moderate width
Operative factors	Width of the flap reduced by: • Excessive resection of the bony hump • Lateral osteotomy too anterior Reduction of the periosteal attachments by wide undermining Internal mucosal tears	Resection of a discreet hump Low osteotomy and impacted fracture An impacted, self-retaining fracture Irregular fracture line Limited undermining

into the nasal fossa, because once mobilised the bony flap is essentially maintained only by its periosteal and mucosal attachments.

Classically, it is said that during the coming together of the bony flaps, an increase in projection of the bony bridge (push up) can be obtained. This occurs in wide noses with a flat bridge; it is unfortunately not the case, as we have seen, in cases where the nasal bones do not rest upon a sufficient bony platform because of the mobilisation of the walls. Rather, it is the contrary which is observed, that is, a slight recoil of the bony flaps which is sometimes not noticed until several months after the operation.

It is therefore indicated at the end of the opera-

tion to resect another 1–2 mm from the septum to prevent a secondary midline projection. The increase in projection is only noted in noses which are not particularly wide with large bony flaps and with a good impaction of the bone superiorly. Table 2.1 summarises the factors which, after a lateral osteotomy and medial luxation, ensure the stability of the bony flap or on the contrary, act against it.

MEDIAN OSTEOTOMY (Fig. 2.51)

The median osteotomy is not always done, particularly if an osteotomy with an 'ascending curve' is performed.

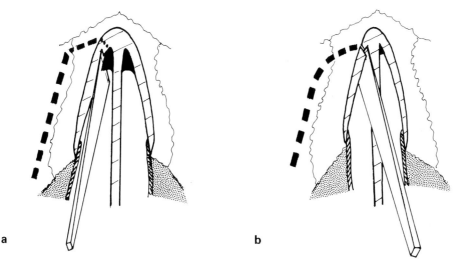

a   b

Fig. 2.51 Median osteotomy. **a.** The osseous corner should be resected: The osteotome is placed flush with the nasal bone with a slight inward orientation. **b.** Narrow root: the osteotome is placed flush with the septum, with a slight orientation outwardly; resection of the osseous corner is not considered.

It is preferable to carry it out before the lateral osteotomy; in effect, the median osteotomy extends the zone of continuity between the lateral osseous flap and the septum (represented superiorly by the nasal spine of the frontal bone and the perpendicular plate of the ethmoid). It creates a *zone of weakness* in the area where one carries out the high fracture by in-fracture.

It is done with a straight, 10 mm-wide osteotome which is placed laterally along the superior portion of the septum, and then impacted vertically towards the nasal spine of the frontal bone. The characteristic change in sound indicates the penetration of the instrument into the denser bone, which is the point at which to stop the progression of the osteotome:

— If the osseous corner needs to be resected (Fig. 2.51a), it is preferable to leave it attached to the septum by placing the osteotome flush with the bone itself for a slight orientation medially.
— On the other hand, if the root is narrow or if one does not see the need for a resection of the osseous corners, the osteotome is placed flush with the septum with a slight orientation laterally (Fig. 2.51b).

LATERAL OSTEOTOMY

1. Sites

These are carried out at the base of the osseous pyramid, that is, along the plane of the anterior surface of the maxilla, and therefore the level of the nasal process of the maxilla. The osteotome passes in front of the lacrimal crest and reaches the root of the nose.

2. Technique

The mucosal incision (Fig. 2.52). A retractor pulls the foot of the ala superiorly, and a short incision is made in the nostril vestibule at a distance and below the intracartilaginous incision; this incision is *like a stab wound*, made with the scalpel in contact with the bone. It is perpendicular with respect to the lateral incision from which it is distinctly separated. It is located just *outside* the lateral border of the piriform orifice, where the retractor engages.

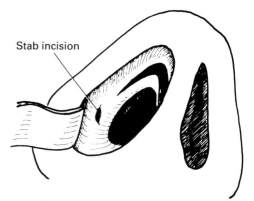

Fig. 2.52 Stab incision permitting passage of a guarded osteotome.

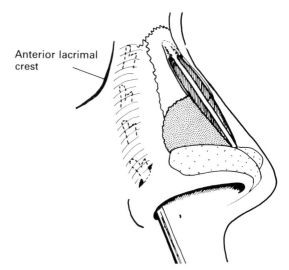

Fig. 2.53 Subperiosteal undermining and path of the osteotome: slightly outward, vertically, then slightly inward.

Subperiosteal undermining (Fig. 2.53). From this incision, the end of a narrow Joseph elevator is introduced, coming into contact with the inferior portion of the lateral border of the piriform orifice which is stripped subperiosteally on both its medial and lateral surfaces, and is thus well marked.

A narrow subperiosteal tunnel is carried out by progression of the elevator which ascends, staying in contact with the bone and moves towards the anterior lacrimal crest, guided by a finger of the other hand so that it stays in front of the lacrimal crest.

This tunnel should be narrow: it should be kept separate from the dorso-nasal undermining by a zone where the periosteum remains attached to the osteocartilaginous segment, which prevents it from falling into the nasal fossa (Fig. 2.50).

The osteotomy. This is carried out with a narrow, guarded osteotome. The guarded portion, placed outwardly under the skin, both permits control of the progress of the osteotome, and avoids damaging skin or mucosa.

This osteotome should be well *sharpened* and have a dove-tail cutting edge permitting constant impaction of the instrument into the bone during its progress.

While one hand firmly holds the osteotome, the assistant taps with a mallet on command from the operator; at the same time, the other hand carefully follows the progress of the instrument by feeling the end of the guard tunnelling under the skin.

The osteotomy is easy in the inferior portion where the bone is thin; as it reaches the superior portion, the thickness is greater, and is noted by a change in sound and a slower progress of the instrument.

The osteotomy is bilateral; it should be strictly symmetrical, which requires a great deal of care in the execution of this important stage.

The direction of the instrument should describe a slight curve, at first superiorly and laterally, then superiorly, to curve upwardly and inwardly in the upper portion, thus following the curve of the bone (Fig. 2.53).

HIGH LUXATION FRACTURE

It remains only to abolish, by fracture, the last line of resistance, which involves the upper portion of the nasal bone.

The site of the high fracture is situated a little below the naso-frontal suture, at the level of the medial canthus. In the case of a classical lateral osteotomy, the high fracture takes place at the superior limit of the bony corners.

In cases where the root of the nose is not too wide (Fig. 2.54a), the medial luxation of the bony flap can be performed by pressure on the nose between the thumb and index finger. The luxation should be simple and occur without resistance, sometimes with a slight cracking sound which signals the high fracture.

In the case of a wide root (Fig. 2.54b), one should extend the zone of continuity between the nasal bone and the septum, by resecting with a narrow rongeur the small bony triangles which constitute a supero-medial bony resistance, preventing on each side the bringing together of the bony segments.

If, in spite of the resection of these bony corners, the luxation still does not take place, one must check the lateral osteotomies and carry out an **out-fracture** by use of a straight osteotome; this passes into the nasal spine, and permits the displacement of the bony flap, the completion of the fracture and the resection of the bony 'corners' (Fig. 2.55). It is only rarely necessary, when the bone is very thick and when the high fracture does not occur in spite of an **out-fracture**, that one will need to complete the fracture by a cutaneous approach, using a narrow 2–3 mm osteotome, after a very small incision at the level of the root of the nose.

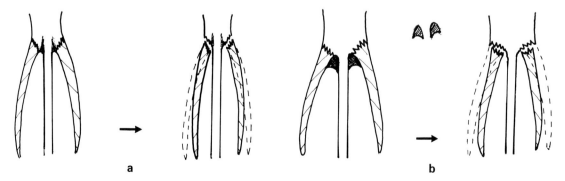

a	b

Fig. 2.54 High fracture. **a.** Root not very wide: the osseous corners are not resected. **b.** Wide root: resection of the osseous corners and high fracture.

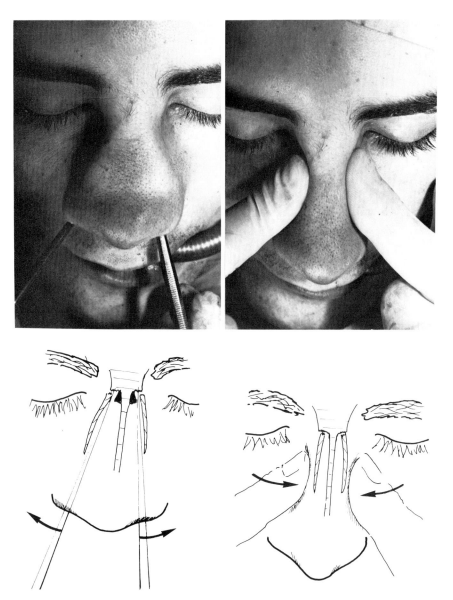

Fig. 2.55 Outward luxation of the bony flaps: resection of the osseous corners and inward luxation of the bony flaps ('in-fracture').

VARIATIONS

The instrument used can be a Joseph saw with a step handle (one needs a right and a left one) the advantage of which is to make the section low. The saw can be used alone, or precede the passage of an osteotome which has then only to follow the groove begun by the saw.

The use of the saw is indicated in post-traumatic noses where there is a risk of opening up multiple fractures with an osteotome, but saws are difficult to use and they are tiring!

Technique used with the saw:

— The saw is introduced by a small saw guide.
— The work is done by the end of the instrument, which saws from above to below.
— Bony debris is removed with a sucker or a curette.

The osteotomy can be carried out through a vestibulo-buccal approach; this is indicated in noses with narrow nostrils, where a further incision will leave a scar and possibly a small adhesion.

It is also indicated in post-traumatic noses, where one needs to resect a thick lateral callus (Aubry-Sénéchal).

The endobuccal incision is made just above the apex of the canine tooth. The following stages are then identical. The only inconvenience of the endobuccal approach rests in the possible occurrence of a hypoaesthesia of the upper lip.

The osteotomy can be carried out by the transcutaneous route. Certain experienced surgeons prefer to use the osteotome through an external approach (using a very narrow, 2–3 mm osteotome), finding this more precise: The lateral osteotomy is done by several osseous 'punctures'. The median osteotomy can separate the root from the rest of the nasal pyramid, and permit en bloc immobilisation of the nose by a high fracture of the septum, which may be useful in deviated narrow noses.

The submucosal osteotomy. One can carry out the osteotomy after undermining not the lateral surface but the medial surface of the maxilla by a submucosal approach. One uses here a very narrow (3–5 mm) osteotome; this has the advantage of avoiding palpebral ecchymoses, which are sometimes considerable.

Location of the osteotomy line. For most authors, the lateral osteotomy should be very low, that is, beginning at the infero-lateral portion of the piriform orifice, extending to the zone immediately in front of the lacrimal crest, a small projection easily identifiable by palpation.

Some surgeons recommend an osteotomy which also begins very low, as in the classical osteotomy, but use a curved osteotome which makes it possible to carry out an osteotomy which in its upper portion describes a curve and approaches the dorsum: This is the 'low to high' osteotomy of Sheen, which one may call an 'ascending curve' (Fig. 2.56). Thus, the non-fractured segment remains very narrow, which permits an easy medial luxation, with a complete, or sometimes 'greenstick', fracture. This fracture occurs at the weak point below the root of the nose, that is, immediately below the osseous 'corners' which it is not necessary to resect. The value of this osteotomy is that it carries out not a translation but a rotation of the bony flaps around the point of the high fracture, which has the advantage of conserving the continuity of the supraorbital lines (Sheen).

This osteotomy is indicated in noses with a narrow root, and when the resection of the bony dorsum is moderate.

PITFALLS OF OSTEOTOMY

An excessive mucosal incision risks creating an adhesion in this zone, where the respiratory equilibrium can be easily interfered with; in fact, it is often the introduction of the osteotome which causes the enlargement of the incision.

A lateral osteotomy which is too anterior risks having the nasal bones fall into the nasal fossae,

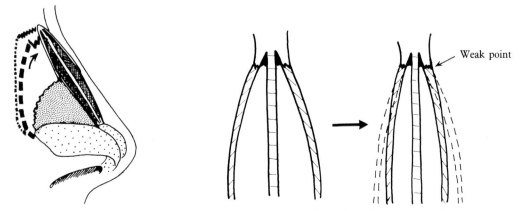

Weak point

Fig. 2.56 Different types of lateral osteotomy: classical lateral osteotomy (dotted line); 'ascending curve' osteotomy (dashed line).

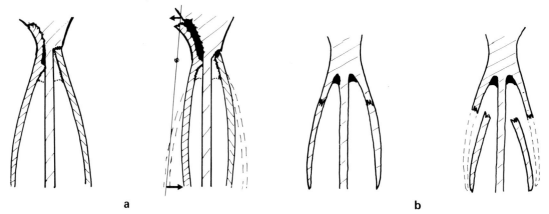

Fig. 2.57 Hazards of the lateral osteotomy. **a.** Fracture excessively high and projection of the bone superiorly by tilting of the bony flap over an inadequately resected corner (rocker formation of Becker). **b.** Fracture too low.

with a resultant pinched nose with a stairstep deformity. When this occurs, the osteotomy should be redone at a lower level, using a fine osteotome. The presence of periosteal adherences, due to limited undermining, makes it possible in this case to maintain the bony fragments in correct position.

An asymmetry between the osteotomy lines sometimes causes a discreet asymmetry of the nose. Greater precision can be obtained in making the osteotomy lines by using a narrow osteotome and carrying out a series of perforations 'en coin' made from *above to below*; the osteotomy is easily completed from *below to above* and follows the line of the perforations; this manoeuvre practically assures symmetry. It takes a little longer, but is very useful for the beginner.

The high fracture, which occurs at the weak point, at the level of the canthus, can be carried out by simple pressure; but sometimes, this fracture does not occur at the proper level (Fig. 2.57). It may be:

— too high, caused by an excessively deep penetration of the osteotome, and involves a medial displacement of the bony flap whose upper extremity then projects outwards. This can be explained by a tilting of the bony flap over a corner which has been inadequately resected; this external bony projection should be corrected either by resection or by transcutaneous fracture using a fine osteotome, after verifying that the bony corner has been correctly resected (Fig. 2.57a)

— too low, the fracture of the bony flap risks causing a localised lateral depression. The insertion of a fragment of the perpendicular plate of the ethmoid, straddling the fracture line, can avoid this deformity (Fig. 2.57b).

INDICATIONS FOR OSTEOTOMY

- *Should one do a lateral osteotomy in all cases?*
- *What type of osteotomy?*
- *Should one do an out-fracture? A resection of the osseous corners?*

1. Indications for the lateral osteotomy

The lateral osteotomy should be performed in most cases. *Before the operation*, a careful examination should note:

— The width of the root of the nose and that of the bony vault, compared with the width of the adjacent cartilaginous bridge.
— The degree of curvature of the nasal bone in both the vertical and transverse directions, certain noses having a marked curvature of the posterior portion of the bony flap. The reduction of the bridge should in these cases be more conservative, because narrowing is difficult to achieve.
— The height: The nasal bones are often very short, the hump being essentially cartilaginous (Fig. 2.58).

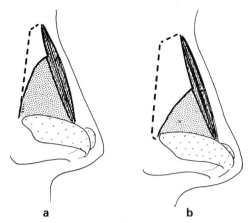

a   **b**

Fig. 2.58 Osteocartilaginous flap with: **a.** short bone; **b.** bone of normal length.

— the direction of the lower border of the nasal bones in the region adherent to the triangular cartilage. An almost horizontal lower border requires that the osteotomy is begun as low down as possible and is directed slightly outward before passing upwards again in order to obtain a good osteocartilaginous flap.

These varied facts may either bring one to perform an osteotomy or not; but in certain cases, it is only after *the reduction of the nasal bridge* that this decision is made.

The osteotomy is not indicated if the nose is very narrow, and if, after lowering of the bridge, there is no flat ledge; a cartilage graft on the dorsum may then be indicated.

In an augmentation rhinoplasty, where a cartilage graft must be placed on the dorsum of a nose of average width, the nose appears less wide after this augmentation without it being necessary to carry out an osteotomy.

If the nasal bones are very short, the mobilisation of the osteocartilaginous flaps by osteotomy risks causing an exaggerated medial displacement, because of the reduced surface of this flap which is essentially cartilaginous. This can result in a pinching in the middle portion of the nose. This phenomenon is aggravated when the osteotomy is not sufficiently posterior, and when the skin is very thin.

The length of the nasal bones has a particular importance because of their role in the support of the osteocartilaginous flap.

When the nasal bones are short, a lateral osteotomy risks weakening the bony support of this flap, with a risk of collapse against the septum.

An osteotomy is indicated in all other cases: wide noses, deviated noses and narrow noses with a large hump.

2. What type of osteotomy to do?

— In the case of a nose of average width with a discreet hump and a normal root, a low to high osteotomy, with an 'ascending curve' is indicated (Fig. 2.56), because, thanks to a high greenstick fracture, or with minimal displacement, it permits an osteotomy that tilts, the bony flap pivoting around the line of the high fracture. In this case, the median osteotomy is not absolutely indispensable, but it can be done with a discreet outward orientation to facilitate the fracture-luxation. As for the resection of the bony corners, this is not necessary since, on the one hand, they are quite small and, on the other hand, the high fracture takes place just below them.

— In the case of a wide nose with or without a hump; it is absolutely necessary to carry out a classical, low lateral osteotomy, permitting a translation medially of the osseous flap which provides the overall narrowing of the nose.

Resection of the bony corners is necessary here, since there exists a risk of a low fracture and insufficient medial luxation. This is facilitated by a median osteotomy with a slight inward orientation (Fig. 2.51a).

3. When should one do an 'out-fracture'?

Then 'out-fracture' can be carried out at the beginning to break the resistance of the osseous bulwark.

But the 'out-fracture' is more indicated when the medial luxation of the bony flap does not take place; in this case, having verified that the lateral osteotomy has been correctly performed, the bony flap is luxated laterally by using an osteotome, and the residual small bony triangles, which form a corner interfering with the coming together of the two flaps, are resected with a rongeur.

4. Resection of the osseous corners

This is necessary every time that the medial luxation of the bony flaps proves insufficient, and in cases where one wants to narrow the upper portion of the nasal bone (J. Oulié).

ALAR CUTANEOUS RESECTIONS

A rhinoplasty is an operation which leaves no visible exterior scar in the majority of cases. In effect, after the reduction of the osteocartilaginous framework, the excess cutaneous cover adapts itself to the underlying osteocartilaginous skeleton, thanks to the elasticity of the skin.

This retraction is made possible by the undermining carried out along the nasal bridge and the tip of the nose, but it is variable, depending on the elasticity and the thickness of the skin. This explains why the reduction should be moderate in an older patient, or in patients with thick skin. On the other hand one may see a temporary shortening when nothing has been done to bring this about.

The cutaneous excess can manifest itself in a number of ways, and if something needs to be done on the skin, it should not be done until the end of the operation.

MODIFICATIONS OF THE NASAL ALAE

Corrections carried out on the nasal alae are often judged necessary, and constitute the last stage of the operation. This is the only time during the operation that anything is done on the exterior cutaneous portion which will thus leave an external scar; this is almost always extremely discreet, because it is situated in the alo-genial fold. The patient should always be informed beforehand.

Resection of the alae is not a physiological operation. It interferes with the musculature of the nasal orifice which plays a role in respiration and also in expression; it should not be undertaken except after careful study noting particularly the dimensions of the nostril orifices which do not always correspond to the excess spread of the nasal ala.

Corrections may be carried out on the nasal alae under three different circumstances:

1. They are often foreseen during the preoperative analysis in cases of a broad nose with thick alae, and in cases of ptosis of the inferior nostril border.

2. At other times, these modifications are not decided upon until the end of the operation: After a reduction, even moderate, of the tip of the nose, one can see a nostril which is more open, a spreading of the foot of the nasal ala which is all the more visible because of the shortening which has been carried out.

3. In certain cases (in particular if one has forgotten to inform the patient), one hesitates to carry out this modification; it is possible to do it later under local anaesthesia.

Seen from an inferior view, the nasal ala has two portions (Fig. 2.59):

— One anterior, supported by the lateral crus
— The other posterior, which corresponds to the foot of the nasal ala, is thick, essentially cutaneous and not containing cartilage. It often has a change in direction from the preceding portion, and this is particularly evident in the Negroid nose.

At the junction of these two portions, there exists on the outer surface an alar depression which is marked to a greater or lesser extent and runs obliquely from below to above (Fig. 2.60). The secondary flattening with reduction of the tip of the nose depends on several factors and varies according to the pre-eminence of these factors. *Anatomical factors:*

— An ala already a bit spread, with a marked alar depression
— An inferior border of the lateral crus that rises almost vertically as it goes back.

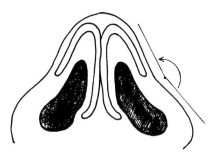

Fig. 2.59 The orientation of the nasal ala changes at the alar groove.

Operative factors:

— The resection of the domes, which facilitates the sliding backwards of the lateral crura towards the mucosa

— The liberation and the resection of the tail of the lateral crura which accentuates a pre-existing alar depression.

Examination in profile. The lower border of the nostril is slightly concave inferiorly in its anterior half, and slightly convex in its posterior half. It should leave the columella visible, but not too much so (Fig. 2.60).

Alae which are too long (Fig. 2.61) require a crescent-shaped cutaneous resection of the lateral portion of the foot of the nasal ala which

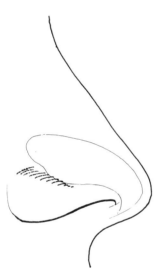

Fig. 2.60 The alar depression or groove.

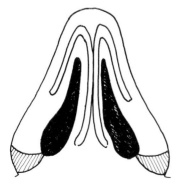

Fig. 2.61 Long alae: the resection is carried out at the base of the nasal ala.

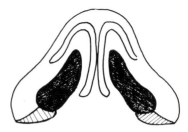

Fig. 2.62 Flattened nose: the resection is carried out at the level of the nostril sill.

extends up into the alo-genial crease; the posterior edge of the excision flush with the alo-genial crease; the width of the excision rarely exceeds 5 mm and is a function of the length of the nasal ala.

Spreading secondary to reduction of the nasal tip can sometimes be corrected by a discreet (2–3 mm) cutaneous resection of the foot of the ala, going very little laterally and not extending into the nostril sill medially.

Major spreading (Fig. 2.62) (Negroid nose), accompanied by very wide nostril orifices, requires a resection extending particularly into the medial vestibular portion of the foot the nasal ala and extending onto the lateral portion of the nasal ala if the latter is long.

Technique of reduction of the alae

— Having carefully and, above all, symmetrically (if the alae are symmetrical), marked the incision, an infiltration of xylocaine-adrenaline solution is carried out

— The incisions are made slowly and a purely cutaneous crescent is excised

— A discreet undermining of the edges of the wound is carried out with a scalpel in order to facilitate the sutures;

— The edges of the wound are brought together with several non-resorbable interrupted sutures, which are removed on the third or fourth day

— The scars are rarely very visible because they are well hidden in the fold. It is only in cases where there is a major external excision that a straight line can be seen in the alo-genial fold.

A ptosis of the lower border of the nasal ala, and a thick alar border, can be corrected simultaneously by a fusiform cutaneous resection of the

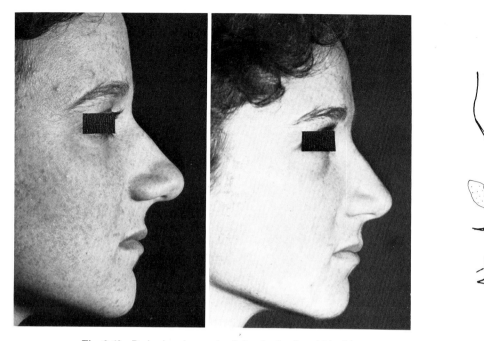

Fig. 2.63 Projecting tip: ptosis of the alar border, thick skin.

— Tip: exteriorisation and resection of the domes (5 mm).
— Triangular shortening.
— Reduction of the cartilaginous and bony bridge with a rasp.
— Lateral osteotomies.
— Resection of the inferior border of the nasal ala corrects the ptosis. Alar base excision (3 mm).

lower border of the nasal ala, a resection which, in frontal view, is an 'inverted V' thus permitting a thinning of the tip of the nose (Figs. 2.63 and 2.64).

— After preliminary marking, the medial incision along the medial portion of the nostril is made, carrying the incision slightly inwardly

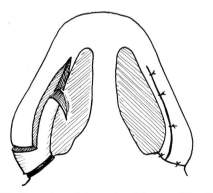

Fig. 2.64 Correction of the ptosis of the nostril border associated with the correction of a long ala.

— two hooks are then placed at the ends of the cutaneous crescent
— The incisions are made orienting the blade of the scalpel in such a way as to remove a V-shaped section; extending to a variable degree into the thickness of the ala;
— The correction of the ptosis of the nostril border can be associated with a resection of the foot of the ala (Fig. 2.64).

CUTANEOUS EXCISIONS (Fig. 2.65)

Apart from the modifications carried out on the nasal alae, external cutaneous resections are rare, but they may be indicated when there is no other way to take care of the cutaneous excess.

The choice between a cutaneous scar and a slight ballooning caused by the skin excess is a difficult one to make.

● In the older subject, a very thin skin with creases and numerous wrinkles has minimal

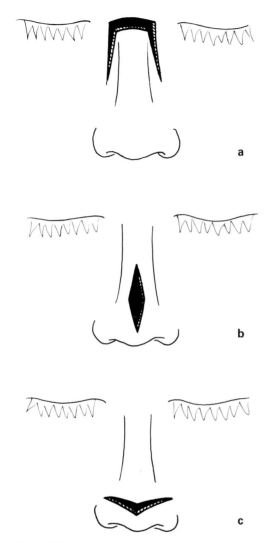

Fig. 2.65 Different types of dorso-nasal cutaneous excision. **a.** In the case of a cutaneous excess in an older patient (R. Peterson). **b.** In the case of a cutaneous excess: thick skin, Polly-beak deformity. **c.** In the case of a very long nose with a falling tip and thick skin.

powers of retraction, and may require a cutaneous 'inverted-V' resection at the root of the nose, assuring the correction of the overly long nose (Peterson's 'open flap rhinoplasty') (Fig. 2.65a).

● During a secondary operation on patients having *thick skin*, a cutaneous excision is indicated:

— In the case of a Polly-beak deformity in a big nose with a wide tip, a vertical fusiform excision centred over the cutaneous excess can in some cases be very beneficial. It reduces the width,

refines the tip and creates a supra-apical depression in place of the Polly-beak deformity (Fig. 2.65b)

— In the case of a very long nose, a horizontal gull-shaped excision carried out in the supra-apical region makes it possible to correct a long nose with a falling tip (Fig. 2.65c).

FINAL CHECKS, TRIMMING AND SUTURE

One inspects the interior and the exterior to be certain of the symmetry of the nose, the regularity of the osteocartilaginous bridge and good nasal airways, and also to be sure that the new osteocartilaginous framework has an anatomy close to normal.

1. On the exterior:

● *Along the midline:* the osteocartilaginous roof should not have any gaps, which would require a check of the osteotomies or the placing of a cartilage graft on the dorsum.

Laterally, the lower border of the triangular cartilage and the upper border of the lateral crus should not present a solution of continuity, which tends to cause the development of a pinched tip or dysfunction of the valve.

● *On the bridge:* one should check for symmetry and look out for irregularities, either projections or depressions.

For this, it is useful to place oneself first above, then below, the patients' head to pick up any discreet deviation, to pass a finger along the bridge, to separate slightly the osseous flaps in order to check that their height is identical, and that the septum does not project with respect to the anterior borders of the nasal bones. The septum should be slightly behind the nasal bones.

The existence of an osseous projection can call for the use of the rasp, holding together the two osseous flaps that were freed by the osteotomy.

A depression can necessitate the insertion of a portion of cartilage or thin bone (perpendicular plate of the ethmoid).

The anterior septal border should be far enough back in its lower third that the tip appears slightly projecting, and when one presses the naso-labial angle firmly against the nasal spine, the profile line

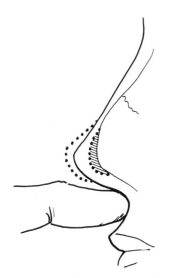

Fig. 2.66 Manoeuvre enabling assessment of an excess of the anterior septal cartilage. Pressure exerted at the level of the foot of the columella causes a drop of the nasal tip. The excess of cartilage is represented by a slight arching above the tip of the nose. This excess should be resected (anterior septal border and anterior border of the triangular cartilages) until the nasal bridge is straight during this manoeuvre. A slight supra-apical saddle depression at the end of the operation is therefore always desirable. Postoperative oedema often causes this to disappear entirely.

should be straight. In effect, after nasal reduction and shortening, the excess skin, particularly if it is thick, tends to create a ballooning above the nasal tip. Removing a bit more septum at this level makes it possible to absorb this cutaneous excess. In the postoperative period, the skin undergoes an inflammatory thickening of varying extent which can last several months and during which one can note, without the septal reduction, an insufficient projection of the tip of the nose which did not appear at the end of the operation (Fig. 2.66).

2. The endonasal examination

Using a speculum or Aufricht retractor, the endonasal examination should verify that the septum is in the midline and is straight (both anterior border and inferior border) and make it possible to see the nasal spine, one surface of which will sometimes require resection (a lateral projection of the spine is often better detected by palpation).

— The inferior septal angle should be rounded.
— The mucosa should not be in excess, in order

to avoid an intranasal fold; a new nasal vestibule should be reconstructed. An excessive projection of the mucosal roof after a resection of the hump should lead one to undermine the septal mucosa a bit more, to allow it to 'recess', and if this is not sufficient, one should conservatively excise the superficial portion of the mucosal roof without completely transecting the mucosa.

— Finally, the patency of the nasal fossae is evaluated by introducing into each nostril a large Killian speculum and checking for the absence of any obstruction, from the nasal spine back to the posterior portion of the septum.

— The integrity of the valve depends on a lateral mucosal and cartilaginous conservation. When the mucosa is in excess, it is resected conservatively; the same is done for the lower border of the upper lateral cartilage where one usually limits oneself to rounding off the medial 'point'.

● *At the level of the tip*: symmetry depends on the remaining cartilages. This can be checked by direct view if there has been a marginal incision; if not, one can make the domes project by pushing up the columella.

Sutures can then be carried out (Fig. 2.67):

● *The use of catgut which dissolves after eight to ten days* has the advantage of not requiring removal of the sutures, which is unpleasant for the patient.

● *The septo-columellar suture* is done first, with three sutures; depending on whether one wants the tip of the nose to project or be slightly retracted, one carries out an orthopaedic suture pushing forward or retracting slightly the columella (Fig. 2.68).

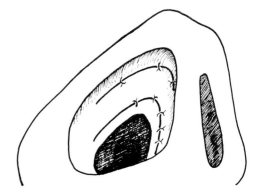

Fig. 2.67   Final sutures.

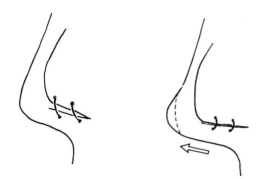

Fig. 2.68 Orthopaedic suture, with a slight anterior projection of the columella.

• *When there is a marginal incision*, it is preferable to place two or three sutures, bringing the edges together without a gap.

• *A suture is done at the level of the dome.*

• *The lateral incision* can be left open if the mucosa is well adapted, otherwise the suture is placed at this level.

• *If the foot of the columella has been resected*, a transfixion suture is carried out with a non-resorbable suture; this suture can be hidden if a resorbable suture is used.

Suture of the mucosal domes. When the nose is very narrow, it is recommended that, after the extramucosal dissection, the mucosal domes are sutured to the anterior septal border with a catgut suture; this constitutes a partial prevention against an eventual pinching of the nasal bridge.

Packing. This is placed after aspirating the nose, and done under direct vision with a speculum. Using packing impregnated with an antibiotic ointment makes it possible to remove the packing without pain or bleeding.

When the marginal incision has been done, the packing is slightly compressive in the vestibule, permitting a good general compression of the 'bucket handle' against the skin of the tip of the nose.

If the septal undermining has been carried posteriorly, the packing will more posterior, making it possible to carefully and gently compress the mucosa against the septum in order to avoid a septal haematoma; this packing is placed along the entire nasal floor.

Finally, in other cases, a moderately compressive packing is placed into each nostril vestibule,

checking particularly that the lateral mucosa has not been forced back.

In a case where a septal deviation has been corrected, the packing may be larger on one side than on the other, in order to provide a selective pressure over several days.

Immobilisation has two aims: to reduce nasal oedema, and to ensure healing after the osteotomies.

Once the packing has been done, adhesive strips 1 cm in width are applied in such a way as to maintain the skin in a 'retracted' position; the tip is similarly maintained by a small adhesive strip passing under the lobule (Fig. 2.69). This 'setting in place' of the skin has an important modelling affect.

A metal splint is then placed on the nose (whatever the material of the splint, plaster or metallic, the important thing is that it be perfectly carried out).

A piece of aluminum 0.7 mm thick is cut with shears, following a pattern previously drawn. The shape of the splint should follow exactly that of the nose, leaving the tip uncovered. The rigidity of metal permits a better lateral retention of the mobilised osseous flaps.

Having protected the edges of the metallic splint, it is placed over the nose, from which it is separated by a surgical dressing. A very effective

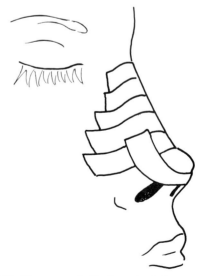

Fig. 2.69 Placement of adhesive strips before immobilisation with a metallic splint.

compression is obtained in the naso-frontal angle area by placing at this level a piece of dressing folded over on itself, upon which several adhesive elastic strips are placed crossways. The splint is then fixed by adhesive elastic strips.

The advantage of the metal splint is:

— To permit a better compression at the level of the naso-frontal angle, where the oedema will be very limited;
— To enable easy removal on the fifth day to check the symmetry of the nose.

The duration of immobilisation with a splint is from 10–12 days. After this period, consolidation has occurred and the oedema greatly reduced. However, it may be necessary to replace the splint at night for one or two weeks, when there is oedema, a wide nose or insufficient consolidation.

POSTOPERATIVE CARE

1. Immediate

Very moderate *bleeding* can sometimes be seen for two or three hours following the operation, but major haemorrhage is very rare.

Oedema and ecchymosis are at their maximum on about the second day and disappear rapidly in 4–5 days; however, subconjunctival ecchymosis can be seen for 2–3 weeks.

The packing is removed:

— The following day if there has been no undermining of the septal mucosa.

— On the third day if the tip has been approached by marginal incisions.
— On the fourth or fifth day if there has been a correction of a septal deviation or an extended mucosal undermining.

• Nasal respiration is poor for several days following removal of the packing and becomes normal in 8–15 days.

• The dressing is removed after the tenth to twelfth day; at this time, the nose has an almost normal appearance and seems a bit shorter than it will eventually appear. In the following weeks everything progressively falls into place; however, in a few rare cases one sees a significant and more lasting shortening, probably associated with a marked retraction of the skin envelope, facilitated by the subperiosteal undermining. A discreet and variable oedema can be seen for several days or weeks.

In certain patients (particularly with dark skin) dark rings under the lower lids can last for several months.

2. Secondary problems

These are sometimes *minimal* with discreet inflammatory phenomena.

On the other hand, these inflammatory phenomena can be very marked for several weeks or months, and require massage and the application of anti-inflammatory creams.

3. Cartilaginous and osteocartilaginous grafts and reimplantations

Grafts are used more and more during secondary rhinoplasties, but equally during primary rhinoplasties.

The advantage of a graft consists in using a fragment of cartilage or bone whose shape is determined beforehand, which permits:

— Either filling a defect
— Or carrying out an anatomical reconstitution of the osteocartilaginous framework permitting a more natural result to be obtained.

The various possibilities are numerous, but it is better to use simple constructions with material harvested in situ (the 'remnants' of the rhinoplasty, and the septum). A good technique makes it possible to avoid possible pitfalls, and to recognise the appearance of new defects.

ON THE GOOD USE OF THE 'REMNANTS'

During a reduction rhinoplasty, the 'remnants' are composed essentially of the following (Fig. 3.1):

— The two fragments from the lateral crura
— And, particularly, the osteocartilaginous hump.

In general, it is better to use fragments previously removed in one piece, which can then be used in many different ways, and in a simpler fashion than can many small fragments which are difficult to put together. This underlines the advantages of the monobloc resection of the nasal hump using an osteotome.

1. The fragments of the lateral crura

These come from the resection of the superior excess of the lateral crura. The pieces of cartilage provided by this are sometimes narrow and fragile and sometimes more substantial.

2. The nasal hump

The nasal hump, removed as a monobloc, that is, with its osseous and cartilaginous portions in continuity, can be used — having been trimmed or cut — for the bridge as well as for the tip of the nose.

THE SEPTUM: HARVESTING SEPTAL CARTILAGE (Fig. 3.2)

Performed after the extramucosal dissection, the shortening, and the reduction of the nasal bridge, the harvesting of septal cartilage can provide a quantity of material larger than one might think, but this requires a correct harvesting technique.

In general, one needs to be able to either take a large piece of a certain dimension, or several fragments from which one can choose.

Technique of septal harvesting

Septal harvesting may be associated with correction of a septal deviation. It is facilitated by the extramucosal dissection, since one can follow the undermining of the septal mucosa posteriorly and down to the nasal floor if one wants to correct a hypertrophic base of the septum or harvest septal bone.

a. An oblique cartilaginous incision is then done 1.5–2 cm behind the anterior septal border.

b. A subperichondrial mucosal undermining along the two sides of the septum is carried out posterior to this incision, using a blunt elevator;

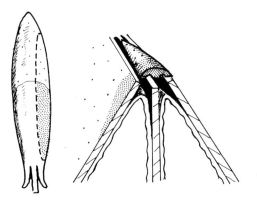

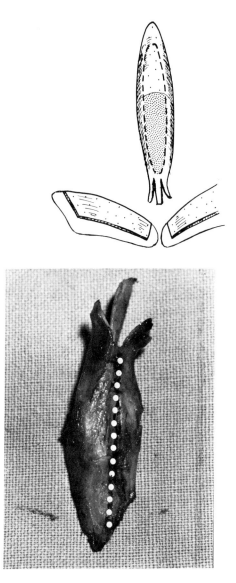

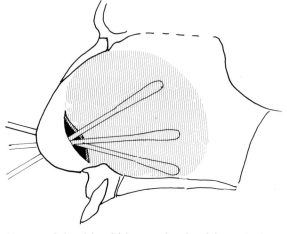

Fig. 3.1 The 'remnants' from a rhinoplasty. Reinsertion of the retailored hump.

— Once the mucosal undermining has been carried out, the two blades of the large Cottle speculum are placed on either side of the septum, and the harvesting can then be done under direct view (with adequate lighting provided by a head mirror or fibre-optic headlight). This harvesting can be partial, or aim to remove the maximum amount of material.

But in all cases, one should preserve a width of 15–20 mm *in front of and above* the anterior and antero-inferior edges of the septum in order not to compromise the stability of the nasal pyramid and

this is generally very easy, but one must be careful when approaching sometimes pronounced projections present at the junction of the septal cartilage with the vomer, where there can be a very projecting ridge covered with a thin and fragile mucosa which tears very easily:

— Undermining is therefore carried out from the nasal spine towards the floor, and then ascends towards the septal cartilage, this makes it possible to avoid tears which in general are of no consequence if they are unilateral.

Fig. 3.2 Subperichondrial mucosal undermining on both sides of the septum behind the septal-cartilaginous incision.

to prevent a global weakening of the septal cartilage with its consequence of a supra-apical 'hatchet cut'.

c. *Large harvesting* (Fig. 3.3).

— An anterior incision going up to the perpendicular plate of the ethmoid is made, obliquely, high up and posterior (this is done with serrated scissors)

— A second cut is made 1.5–2 cm behind the previous one. Then, with flat jawed forceps, a large fragment is harvested, removing in continuity the septal cartilage and the perpendicular plate of the ethmoid. This fragment often has a thickening at the level of the osteocartilaginous junction which is fragile

— The foot of the septum, sometimes hypertrophic, can furnish a bony fragment of a volume which sometimes makes it possible to avoid harvesting from the iliac region; this harvesting is done with a curved osteotome driven along the nasal floor.

d. *Partial harvesting makes it possible to obtain:*

— Either a thick fragment, by changing the direction of harvesting horizontally, towards the base of the septum

— Or a thinner and more regular fragment, by orienting the direction of the harvesting towards

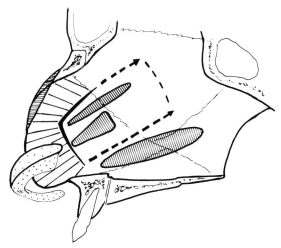

Fig. 3.3 The various possibilities for harvesting a small or large septal graft. In front of the cartilaginous incision is the area to be preserved.

the perpendicular plate of the ethmoid. This flat graft is often thin and can be modelled very easily with serrated scissors — or a graft which is purely cartilaginous;

— Or a mixed graft, whose osteocartilaginous junction is relatively fragile and should be manipulated with caution, particularly during modelling.

Septal adherences

In cases of septal adherences associated with previous surgery on the septum, and as long as there is no respiratory obstruction due to an anterior deviation, harvesting can be carried out through a posterior mucosal incision made on one side, which permits a direct approach to the septum. In fact, the difficulties of harvesting the septal cartilage, can be considerable, and lead to harvesting of the auricular conchal cartilage.

At the end of the operation

At the end of the operation it is advisable to replace between the two undermined mucosal surfaces the cartilage fragments remaining after flattening them by cartilage crushing forceps. In effect, one can observe after a major septal harvesting a respiratory obstruction associated with a 'floating septum', which is mobile during each nasal inspiration and expiration.

— A symmetrical packing fixes the mucosal surfaces properly in place for three to five days.

— The suture of an incision or a tear in the mucosa can be carried out with a resorbable suture; otherwise, the packing should be properly placed over mucosa which has been carefully spread out.

THE AURICULAR CARTILAGE (Fig. 3.4)

It is possible, in cases where harvesting septal cartilage is impossible, to obtain *thicker*, fibro-elastic cartilage, but whose *contour* requires judicious carving.

Technique of harvesting

a. The anterior approach is faster and more simple. Bleeding is greatly reduced but the scar,

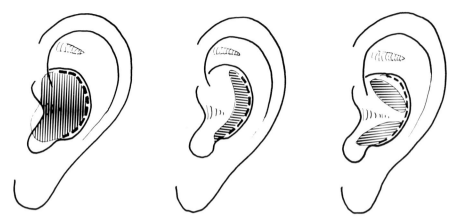

Fig. 3.4 Harvesting from the concha: total or partial.

although it may be very discreet, does not have the advantage of being totally hidden, as is the case with a retro-auricular scar.

After infiltration with xylocaine-adrenaline solution, a cutaneous incision is made at the level of the lateral border of the concha, that is, within the anterior border of the antihelix.

b. The posterior approach has the advantage of a retro-auricular scar. It requires a preliminary establishing of landmarks with needles inserted after first marking them on the anterior slope

— The anterior subperichondrial undermining is easily carried out in both cases using a blunt elevator; it is extended as far as the root of the helix and to the external auditory canal.

— The cartilage is cut at the lateral border of the concha, and the posterior undermining extended far posteriorly. This undermining preserves the posterior perichondrium.

c. The harvesting may be:

● Partial, taken from the lateral concha. This provides a long, regular fragment whose slight curve can be corrected by parallel incisions or by cartilage crushing forceps.

● Total. The fragment obtained is elongated and oval, and has a large surface area. It can be used by rolling it up along its best longitudinal axis and reducing its thickness in certain areas. This rolling-up is maintained by several sutures taken through the perichondrium conserved on the posterior surface. One can thus correct substantial

depressions; the empty spaces are filled with small fragments crushed previously. But the concha can also be used in fragments which are superimposed or used alone, either at the level of the nasal bridge, or that of the nasal tip.

GRAFTS TO THE BRIDGE

1. Choice of graft

● The choice of graft depends on its destination: to fill a gap reinforce a weak structure, or reconstitute the bony roof; but it also depends on the thickness of the skin.

● At the level of the nasal bridge, one can choose:

— Either a fragment of flat, regular septal cartilage of varying length sometimes in continuity with a bony fragment from the perpendicular plate of the ethmoid; this constitutes an excellent graft which can be placed on the nasal bridge;

— Or, the nasal hump, which can be used in various ways.

The reinsertion of the tailored nasal hump (Fig. 3.1), that is, reduced in dimension according to the Skoog's technique (1974).

The osteocartilaginous nasal hump, resected as a one piece fragment, is carefully stripped of all epithelium and small fragments of tissue adhering to both its superficial and deep surfaces. Then, it is tailored either in order to obtain a hump of reduced dimension, or sectioned longitudinally along a vertical paraseptal line, in order to obtain a longer osteocartilaginous fragment.

The advantage of this reinsertion is to close in an anatomical fashion the gap which can exist in the osteocartilaginous roof, in spite of the bringing together of the osteocartilaginous side walls. This reconstitution has the further advantage of providing a regular and natural bridge (Lévignac 1958).

It is important, for the conditions for the reinsertion be satisfactory, that the extramucosal dissection is done without tearing the mucosal lining.

One uses this reinsertion for several reasons:

— Either because the hump has been somewhat excessively resectioned (an error in estimation).
— Or because the resection has been deliberately excessive: in the case of a very large nose, for example, where the reinsertion has been planned before the operation (Fig. 3.5).
— Or in a nose with a strong lateral convexity, because the mobilisation of the walls after the osteotomy leaves a gap superiorly because of the curvatures and it is not desirable to have the skin in direct contact with the mucosa.
— Or in large noses, where after the reduction one notices that the skin does not 'follow', and it is preferable to add the thickness of a graft along the length of the bridge.
— Finally, in certain deviated noses, with an anterior deviation which it is difficult to correct (Fig. 3.6).

At the level of the lateral portions of the nose, thin fragments of the perpendicular plate of the ethmoid or of crushed cartilage can be placed flat, superficially over the osteocartilaginous flap, either to reinforce a weak triangular cartilage or to reestablish symmetry.

2. Shaping the grafts (Fig. 3.7)

When a graft is planned at the level of the bridge, one should always bear in mind the convexity of the osteocartilaginous bridge; one should take account of this when shaping the graft in both the vertical direction and the transverse direction. This leads to the use of elongated, but supple grafts, which, if necessary, are made flexible by superficial incisions. The ends of these grafts are made thinner, and tapered in order to bend in the direction imposed by cutaneous pressure. The surface of the grafts should be regular, smooth, and rounded in a transverse direction to avoid a lateral projection. The osseous ends of the graft are also thinned and curved backwards.

3. The layer of coverage for the graft: the skin (Fig. 3.7)

The nasal skin varies considerably from one patient to another; sometimes it is very thick or, on the contrary, very thin.

A lateral xerographic X-ray shows that the thickness of the skin varies from above to below.

In the upper naso-frontal third, the thickness is 7.5 mm on average, the skin is often thick and the subcutaneous tissue abundant.

In the middle third, that is, overlying the hump, the thickness is reduced to 3 mm on average; and the subcutaneous tissue is greatly reduced but the skin is often fine and very mobile, sliding easily over the osseous framework. This mobility is reduced inferiorly, at the level of the cartilaginous framework.

In the lower third, the skin is thicker and adheres to the muscle and cartilage; the sebaceous glands are more numerous, and the pores appear more dilated.

It is thus over the middle third that the risk of irregularities or of projections is the greatest, so that the graft should be smooth and regular at this level, and extend superiorly and inferiorly towards the regions where the skin is thicker.

An irregularity or projection can sometimes appear quite late (after more than a year); this is more likely if cutaneous atrophy occurs, with thinning of the skin layers.

4. The bed of the graft

This is constituted:

• In its upper half, by the three osseous surfaces (the osseous septum and the nasal bones).

• In its lower half, by three cartilaginous surfaces (the septum and the upper lateral cartilages).

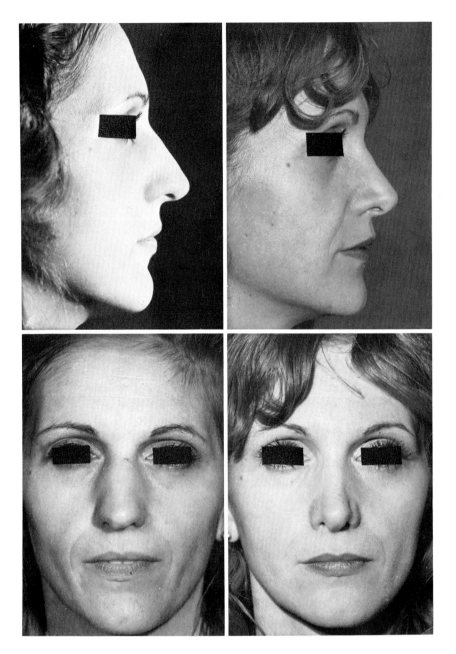

Fig. 3.5 Nose with a wide bridge, wide root and tip, discreet hump and skin of moderate thickness.

— Extramucosal dissection.
— Tip: reduction of the height of the lateral crura and domes (without section).
— Triangular shortening anteriorly, by 3 mm.
— Resection with osteotome of the osteocartilaginous hump.
— Lateral osteotomies, plus resection of the osseous corners followed by an in-fracture.
— Reinsertion of the tailored hump.

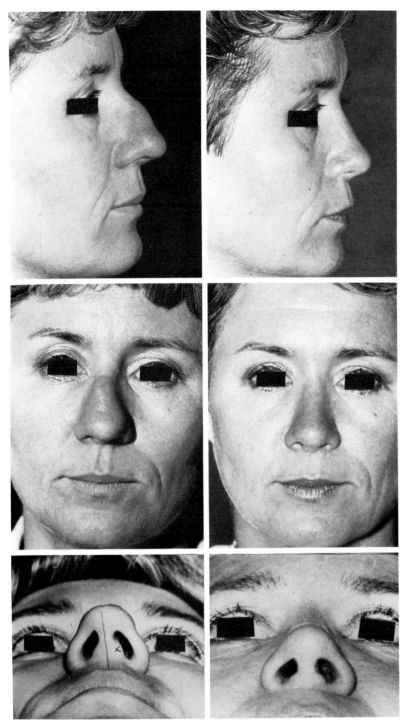

Fig. 3.6 Deviated nose with large hump, thick skin, and wide, projecting tip.

— Extramucosal dissection.
— Tip: reduction of the width by resection of the superior excess of the lateral crura and lowering of the tip by resection of the domes, encroaching slightly on the mesial crura.
— Triangular shortening (2–3 mm anteriorly).
— Resection of the osteocartilaginous hump in slight excess, and repositioning of a lateral fragment of the hump over the nasal bridge.
— Correction of septal deviation, and lateral osteotomies.
— Alae: resection of the alar base (3 mm).

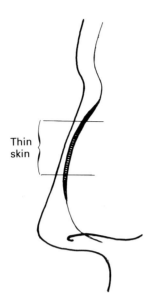

Fig. 3.7 Straight cutaneous profile: The osteocartilaginous profile is slightly convex.

The anterior border of the cartilaginous septum has lost its anterior thickening because of the resection of the hump:

— The graft can be placed as an *inlay*, that is, layered between the two osteocartilaginous flaps, after having moved the septal bridge back by 1–2 mm (Fig. 3.9a).
— We find it more easy and certain to place it as an *onlay*, as is done with reinsertions of the nasal hump; in these cases, it is important that the anterior edges of the osteocartilaginous flaps are at the same level and are smooth and regular, and that the anterior septal border is slightly set back (Fig. 3.9b).

Generally, it is preferable, whether one is dealing with a graft on the bridge or on the tip, that the bed is not excessively large, so that the graft does not 'float'. This is not always possible, and it is important to ensure that the fragments are kept in place.

5. Assemblage of the grafts

The graft may be made up of one single fragment, but it is often necessary, to obtain the desired thickness and volume, to assemble several fragments, bind them together, and then introduce the construction so created (Fig. 3.9).

Several fragments of cartilage can be superimposed (2–3 layers), the fragments becoming more narrow towards the surface (Fig. 3.8). The whole construction is kept together either by transfixing sutures or by encircling sutures; the structure made should have be regular, smooth and rounded, and be thinned out at its extremities. If a rolled-up conchal cartilage is used, the remaining fragments of cartilage should be used to fill the dead spaces.

6. Placement of the grafts.

The grafts are preferably put in place at the end of the operation, before the final sutures. They should be placed in a precise area whose limits have been marked with ink on the skin after a preliminary test placement.

It may be useful to keep the grafts in place by transcutaneous sutures: For this one uses catgut sutures which are held by adhesive strips and are removed very easily on about the fifth day. With a modelling dressing, a perfect adaptation can be assured.

A preliminary suture of the mucosal domes by one or two sutures has two aims:

— It permits a better seating of the graft (Fig. 3.9a).
— It maintains the triangular cartilages and prevents their collapse against the septum.

GRAFTS TO THE NASAL TIP

Cartilaginous grafts of the tip of the nose have been used particularly in secondary rhinoplasty; their use has become more frequent in primary rhinoplasty, where their role is different and consists of assuring a better support and better projection of the tip of the nose, only noses with a very short columella (the Negroid nose in particular) benefit from cartilage grafts.

Among the manoeuvres which contribute to the loss of nasal tip projections during rhinoplasty, certain involve the *alar cartilages* (Fig. 1.17):

— Resection of the domes, particularly if it involves the medial crura.
— Reduction of the height of the lateral crura.
— Resection of the tail of the lateral crura.

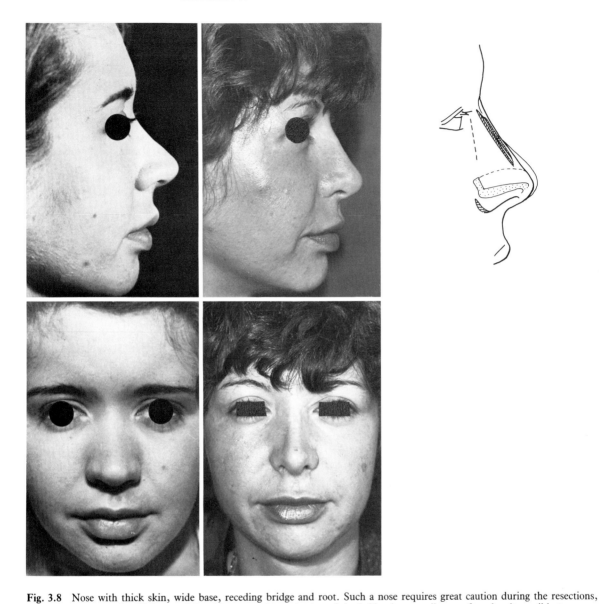

Fig. 3.8 Nose with thick skin, wide base, receding bridge and root. Such a nose requires great caution during the resections, taking into account the thickness of the skin cover; the projection of the bridge by a cartilage graft makes it possible to carry out a moderate reduction of the tip.

— Very limited subperiosteal undermining.
— Extramucosal dissection.
— Tip: reduction of the superior excess of the lateral crura.
— Lowering by 4–5 mm of the cartilaginous bridge.
— Lateral osteotomies.
— Cartilage grafts (septal) in three layers, placed on top of each other and held together by two non-resorbable sutures.
— Alar resections (3 mm).

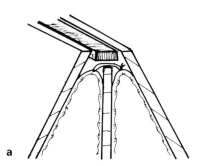

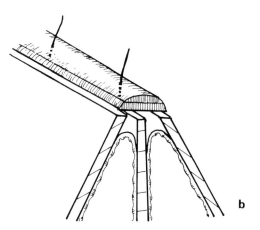

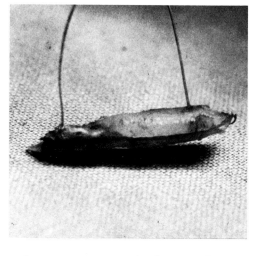

Fig. 3.9   Bed of the graft. **a.** Built-in graft. **b.** Grafts placed as 'onlay': two cartilage fragments, one placed on top of the other. The grafts are held in place by two sutures transfixing the grafts and the skin.

But *other manoeuvres* can also have a role:

— The intersepto-columellar transfixion incision, particularly when it is extended towards the nasal spine.
— Resection of the cartilaginous bridge, because the reduction of the volume of the cartilaginous framework immediately creates an excess of skin coverage which is not supported by the septal strut, and the height of which acts on the tip of the nose.
— Resection of the nasal spine, on which rests the feet of the mesial crura.

During a rhinoplasty, the aim is to obtain a balanced relationship between the level of the projection of the tip of the nose, and that of the nasal bridge; in fact, one always seeks to obtain a projection of the tip such that the bridge is slightly set back, in order to avoid the unsightly appear-ance of a rounded tip. Thus, it is recommended *to begin with surgery of the nasal tip* in all cases where the latter poses a problem (very projecting tip, re-tracted tip, round tip, flabby tip, thick skin). In these cases, the level of the nasal profile will be determined taking account of the projection of the nasal tip.

1. Indications for a graft may be established:

a. Before the operation:

• *In noses with a flabby tip.* These are noses which often have a rounded tip, the skin some-times rather thick and without any visible cartilaginous projection. Palpation shows the flab-biness, the lack of spring of the tip of the nose; the cartilaginous borders are not perceptible through the skin, as they are in certain tips with a visible cartilaginous relief.

At operation, one often finds soft cartilages, lacking elasticity, which are not very thick and which are difficult to dissect.

In these cases, it is preferable to place a cartilage graft which has, in particular, a *role in providing support* and a framework for the tip of the nose, rather than providing projection. However this graft serves to limit the loss of projection which is more marked without the graft, and to avoid a rounded tip postoperatively.

• *In Negroid noses*, where the nose appears wide and with a flat bridge, the point is round, the skin thick and the columella short; the alae are flattened, with a break at the height of the alar crease.

The placement of the grafts should be carried out along the entire extent of the nasal bridge, which contributes to project slightly the tip of the nose by reducing the 'weight of the skin', but grafts are also placed at the level of the columella.

One lengthens the columella thanks to the mobilisation of the nasal walls which facilitates sliding. This lengthening cannot be maintained unless one supports the columella with a graft.

• *In noses with a bulbous tip and thick skin*, it is not rare that reduction of the lateral crura with the aim of reducing the bulbous aspect, diminishes the spring in the projection of the tip which therefore should be reinforced with a cartilaginous graft (Fig. 3.10).

The latter also makes it possible to obtain a better definition of the tip by reliefs which are more marked.

b. At the end of the operation. This, one could say, is a last-minute decision, made if, after surgery of the tip and lowering of the bridge, the projection of the nasal tip is still not satisfactory.

In these cases, if the resection of the hump has been substantial, and if the skin is thick, it is preferable to augment the projection of the nasal tip with a graft, rather than to lower the bridge, particularly in the case of a wide nose.

2. Materials to use

One may choose between:

— The osteocartilaginous hump whose osseous and cartilaginous portions can furnish an adequate graft by a transverse section.
— The septum, when it is preferable to have large and thick fragments.
— The conchal cartilage, which can be favoured for the thickness and rounded form of the cartilage which is provided.

3. Which procedure to use?

There are numerous procedures, each of which has an indication depending on the defect to be corrected, the thickness of the skin, the quality and dimensions of the harvested graft and, finally, the experience of the surgeon.

The cartilage graft can be placed either over the domes as an *onlay*, or between the mesial crura and the domes, or else beneath the mesial crura and the domes.

Whatever the procedure, one should above all avoid exchanging one defect for another: in effect, the placement of a cartilage graft in the area of the nasal tip can bring about, if one does not take care, a deformity or cartilaginous projections which are even more visible when the skin is thin.

a. The 'fleur de lys' of Tessier (Fig. 3.11). This is a logical and anatomical procedure which uses a thick, rectangular septal fragment 15–20 mm long and 5 mm wide. This fragment is split sagittally with a scalpel at one of its ends over a length of 5—7 mm, so as to obtain two 'petals' which, pulled apart, have the appearance of a fleur de lys. This graft is introduced between the two mesial crura, the two petals resting over the domes. One can also use two fragments of lateral crura added to one of the ends.

The inconvenience of the procedure rests in the midcolumellar cutaneous incision made over the apical columellar segment. The scar is almost invisible but may not be accepted by the patient.

We prefer to place this fleur de lys through a marginal incision, when necessary guiding the 'petals' by a catgut suture leaving at the level of the domes (Fig. 5.24).

The fleur de lys is a good procedure for the asymmetric tips of cleft-lip noses, and when one has available a thick fragment of cartilage.

b. The Jost graft (Fig. 3.12). This combines a sagittal support graft fixed to the nasal spine, therefore above the mesial crura, with a modelling graft slid beneath the mesial crura; a non-absorbable suture joins the two fragments and prevents the upper fragment from sliding superiorly during scar formation.

This is a procedure useful in very short columellas (Negroid nose, and secondary rhinoplasty).

c. The onlay graft (Peck) (Fig. 3.13). One uses a fragment, or often two fragments of cartilage (preferably cartilage harvested from the auricular concha), which are placed transversely above the domes with fixation provided by two trans-

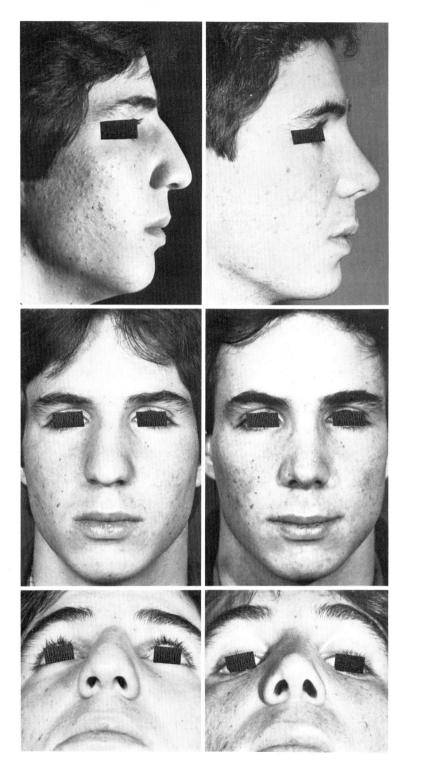

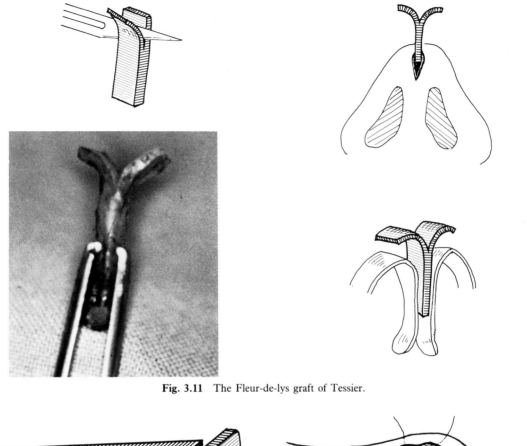

Fig. 3.11 The Fleur-de-lys graft of Tessier.

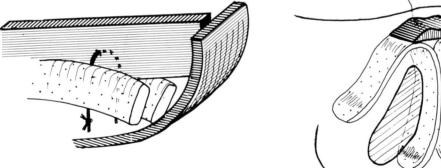

Fig. 3.12 The Jost graft.

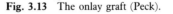

Fig. 3.13 The onlay graft (Peck).

Fig. 3.10 Nose with a projecting root, discreet hump, tip slightly receding, skin a little thick. Although discreet, the necessary lowering of the nasal bridge, in this type of nose involves a diminution of the projection of the tip which needs to be compensated for by a graft.

— Extramucosal dissection.
— Triangular shortening (3 mm anteriorly).
— Tip: reduction of the superior excess of the lateral crura, followed by staggered incisions over the domes (after exteriorisation).
— Resection of the osteocartilaginous hump extending into the root.
— Lateral osteotomies and resection of the osseous corners.
— Cartilage graft to the tip of the nose by a graft of triangular shape taken from the septum, introduced through a marginal incision and held in place by a transcutaneous catgut suture (Sheen).

cutaneous sutures coming out through the domes and tied over a pledget. This is a simple procedure which is indicated if one has only small fragments of cartilage.

d. Sheen's procedure (Figs 3.14 and 3.10). Sheen has emphasised the usefulness of cartilage grafts in primary rhinoplasty, to augment the projection of the tip of the nose in those cases where the desired equilibrium favours this solution rather than further lowering of the bridge, which is constant with a more conservative approach to surgery.

The Sheen procedure is not easy and requires, on the one hand, a graft of very good quality and of well-defined dimensions, and on the other hand a very careful technique.

It is preferable to use septal cartilage, but a fragment of septal bone or nasal hump, can also provide a good graft. By good graft, one means a thick graft, not weakened by fractures, sufficiently long and of a width that varies, depending on the appearance of the skin and its suppleness.

A marginal incision is made on the side of the operator as far as the apico-columellar junction which marks the inferior limit of the pocket for the graft.

This pocket is created with scissors or a scalpel, and should be made so that the graft should not be too difficult to introduce, nor too easy.

The graft is introduced a first time into its pocket to assess its length: if the projection under the skin is excessive, one shortens it slightly and a V-shaped notch is made in its narrowed posterior extremity; this notch is intended to limit the vertical displacement.

Once in place, the graft should be orientated at 30–35° to the horizontal.

It is preferable to fix the graft by two catgut sutures which come out through the columella and which are kept in place by adhesive strips.

The sutures of the marginal incisions are carefully performed at the end of the operation.

The length of the graft is difficult to determine: too short, and it does not provide the desired projection; too long, and it can project under the skin and this is bothersome, particularly if the skin is thin. A cartilaginous projection may also be seen at the apico-columellar junction. When the graft goes posterior to the apico-columellar junction, this can result in a flat appearance of the inferior lower border of the columella.

Displacement of the graft can occur if the pocket is too large and if the marginal incisions have been made.

e. The 'swallow' graft (G. Aiach) (Fig. 3.15). The nasal hump, resected as one piece, can provide a cartilaginous graft whose 'swallow' shape has the advantages of the Peck procedure and of

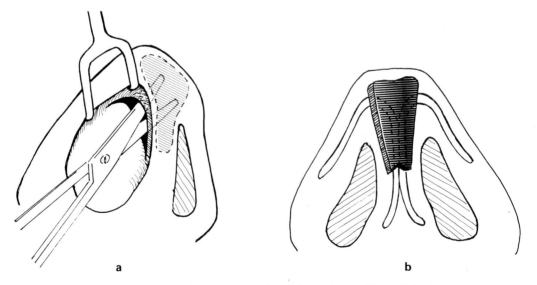

a   b

Fig. 3.14 Sheen's procedure. **a.** Preparation of the pocket. **b.** The graft in place.

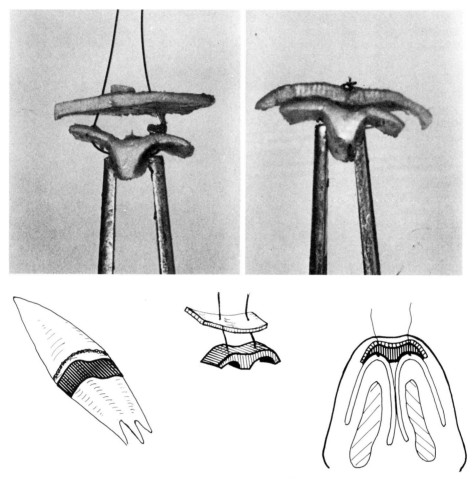

Fig. 3.15 The 'swallow graft' (G. Aiach).

the fleur de lys. This graft is taken from the upper portion of the cartilaginous hump by two horizontal cuts 5 mm apart. The transverse section shows that, at this level, the septum broadens out and joins with the triangular cartilages through a dense, solid and supple fibrous connection. The inferior surface of the graft is concave on either side of the septum and rests on the domes, while the middle septal portion passes between the two domes.

The superficial surface of the graft has a medial depression which is limited laterally by the two lateral projections of the two lateral projections of the two lateral portions of the dorsal septum, projections which give the dome a natural appearance.

The placement of the graft is done through a marginal route after undermining between the two domes and over their superficial surface. The median septal portion of the graft is placed between the domes and the two 'alae' are guided by a thread coming out through the domes.

The advantages of this graft are, on the one hand, that it has good, natural contours on its superficial and deep surfaces without any further modification being necessary; and, on the other hand, the suppleness of the lateral expansions destined to project the domes. One can add a fragment of the lateral crus to augment the thickness.

4. What factors come into play in the choice of a procedure?

a. The projection of the tip of the nose. A

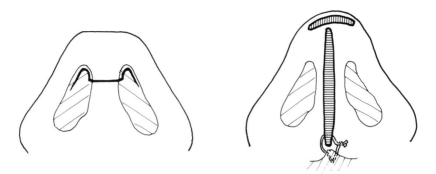

Fig. 3.16   The Rethi incision and the 'parasol' graft.

very short columella is an indication for placing between the two mesial crura a columellar strut fixed to the nasal spine posteriorly; this strut should, if one wants to avoid a cutaneous projection, be associated with a conchal graft; the entire assemblage has the shape of a parasol. The Rethi incision permits, in these cases, an excellent approach at the price of a minimal scar (Fig. 3.16).

When the columella is of normal length, one can choose between the Sheen procedure, if one wants to improve the profile of the columella, or an *onlay* graft.

b. The use of the 'swallow' graft depends on having a cartilaginous hump taken in one piece and having thick cartilage (Fig. 5.5).

c. The appearance of the skin. If the skin is very fine, the slightest irregularity will be associated with a cutaneous projection; one may prefer, if the graft is thin, to place it transversely over the domes or to use a conchal graft whose rounded relief fits perfectly. In general, the area of the graft pressing on the skin should be larger when the skin is fine.

d. The quality of the harvested graft. If one has septal cartilage, an excellent fragment may constitute an indication for the Sheen technique (Fig. 5.22 and 5.23).

On the other hand, if the fragment is too small, or fractured, it may be preferable to use an onlay graft.

e. The preparation of the placement of the graft should be done extremely carefully. The Sheen procedure is more difficult to carry out correctly than an onlay graft which is relatively simple.

The aim of nasal plastic surgery is to obtain a pretty nose, but above all a nose in harmony with the face. This harmony is sometimes seen differently by different surgeons. Certain operators deliberately choose to reduce all noses and to lower the bridge further to obtain a satisfactory projection of the tip of the nose.

The evolution of rhinoplasty towards a more conservative approach, explains the tendency to prefer conserving the continuity of the domes and, in certain cases, projecting the tip of the nose by cartilaginous graft rather than by further reduction of the nasal bridge.

GRAFTS TO THE NASO-LABIAL ANGLE. THE PREMAXILLA

A re-entrant naso-labial angle, and receding premaxilla can be seen in cases of anomalies of the maxilla with malocclusion whose correction should be the obligatory first stage (Fig. 3.17).

When the dental occlusion is normal, one can see numerous anomalies of the naso-labial angle and the premaxilla which require bone or cartilage grafts.

1. The surgical approach

The intersepto-columellar incision extended towards the nasal spine is often adequate, and permits a good approach to the nasal spine. This enables the placement of grafts (the 'remnants' of the septo-rhinoplasty) both opposite the nasal spine and in the area of the premaxilla, that is, the region of the maxilla located at the base of the nose. A

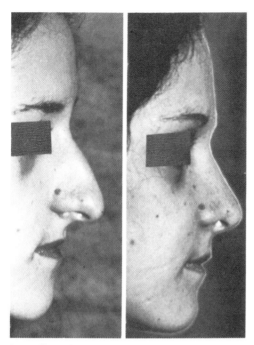

Fig. 3.17 Operative correction in two stages. First stage: advancement of the maxilla by a LeFort I osteotomy. Second stage: rhinoplasty.

pocket is created, either after subperiosteal undermining in the area of the nasal spine, or at the level of the base of the columella where cartilaginous fragments can be placed in a subcutaneous pocket to correct a re-entrant nasolabial angle.

The endobuccal approach is however preferable in major cases, notably when a bone graft is envisaged. The mucosal incision is made in the labial vestibule, making an inverted V-shaped incision in the area of the frenulum of the upper lip. The nasal spine is reached and subperiosteal undermining carried out on both sides. The infero-lateral border of the piriform orifice is filed and undermining of the nasal floor can be achieved by this route, connecting up with the septal undermining which 'provides' mucosa.

When the naso-labial angle is re-entrant, with a degree of maxillary hypoplasia, it is necessary to place a bone graft (harvested from the iliac region, the base of the septal bone, or the nasal bony hump) fixed to the nasal spine and destined either to reconstitute a missing inferior septal border or the nasal spine.

2. The fixation to the nasal spine with a steel wire osteosynthesis

This is very simple and quick, and can be carried out in the following manner: with a square-tipped drill, two perforations, converging posteriorly, are made in the bone; these perforations join posteriorly and thereby permit the passage of a .030 mm wire (Fig. 3.18).

The square-tipped drill can also be used to make perforations in the graft, which help the osteosynthesis.

3. In the case of major maxillary hypoplasia

In this case, flat fragments of spongy bone are placed transversely across the premaxilla in layers (Fig. 3.19).

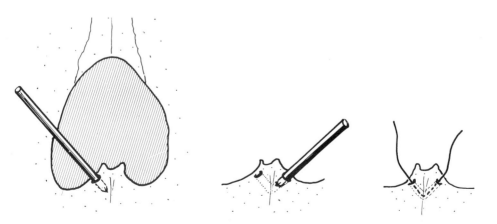

Fig. 3.18 Osteosynthesis of the nasal spine using a thin awl: V-shaped perforations and passage of a wire.

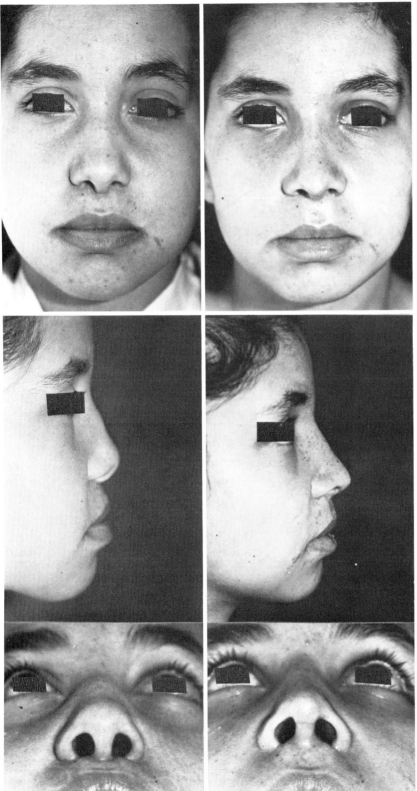

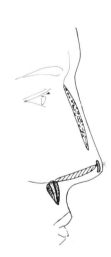

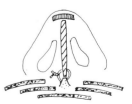

Fig. 3.19   Flattened nose. Maxillary hypoplasia (Binder's syndrome).
— Rethi incision.
— Harvesting of septal cartilage.
— Cortico-cancellous bone graft (iliac) after a freshening of the naso-frontal angle.
— Vestibular buccal incision: three layers of fragments of cancellous bone were placed over the premaxilla on each side of the nasal spine.
— Reduction of the superior excess of the lateral crura.
— Tip: columellar strut (fragment of cortical bone), wired to the nasal spine: cartilage graft over the domes, resting on the columellar strut; suture of the domes.

4. Secondary rhinoplasty

GENERAL COMMENTS

A large variety of defects can be observed following rhinoplasty:

a. Minimal defects, which a patient who is overly demanding and narcissistic wants at all costs to get rid of. In this case, the patient often returns to the surgeon because the overall result is good.

b. Major defects. A nose which is veritably 'ruined' due to lack of experience; the defects are, in these cases often multiple and inter-related, and the patient more willingly consults another surgeon; this explains why, in publications, the major mistakes are always those of others!. . .

c. Between the two. There is an entire range of defects, accepted to a greater or lesser extent, which usually comprise an excessive reduction or, on the contrary, insufficient reduction; this is witness to the precision demanded whenever this delicate operation is performed.

Failures can be due either to a bad choice of operation, an error of technique, or an error of assessment (Fig. 4.1). This last point raises an essential and delicate problem. In effect, a rhinoplasty is one of the rare surgical interventions where technique alone is not sufficient to assure a good result. It is necessary to have a good sense of proportion in three dimensions. But the character itself of this operation, which deals with patients who are sometimes suffering from complex psychological problems, explains why it is difficult, even possessing a cause of form, to satisfy every individual.

Defects may appear immediately after the removal of the dressing, or they may not appear for several months, or even a year. One must try to 'prevent' these minor and major failures and for this reason the surgeon should, during the procedure, take into account each minor detail. With increasing experience, the surgeon becomes more and more demanding of himself.

Does the treatment present particular difficulties? One can encounter, depending on the damage done, serious difficulties aggravated by the psychological effects of lost hope.

The treatment of these sequelae of rhinoplasty should be preceded by a careful *analysis* of the deformities (an analysis which should be carried out before every rhinoplasty).

ANALYSIS

a. The interrogation of the patient should establish:

— The nature of the inital operation. Examination of the original photographs can make it possible to reconstruct the stages.
— Was there a pre-existing nasal or septal deviation?
— Has there been an operation on the septum?
— What was the postoperative course: oedema, circulatory problems, respiratory difficulties, a subsequent deformity.
— After how long a time did the nose become stable?

b. The examination of the nose, and particularly palpation, makes it possible to assess the suppleness of the skin, its thickness, and the existence of a cartilaginous or fibrous Pollybeak deformity, and any cartilaginous or osseous projections.

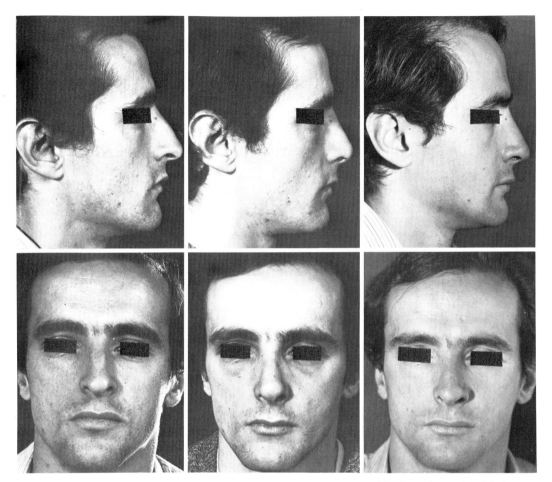

Fig. 4.1   Poorly conceived rhinoplasty. Nose overly reduced (centre), and not accepted by the patient, who wished to return to a nose close to his original nose (left). Augmentation rhinoplasty using a graft (the bony base of the septum in large amounts) over the nasal bridge, and a cartilage graft of the nasal tip (right).

— The existence of cutaneous problems: with a skin which is thin and pale over a cartilaginous or bony projection, a zone of pressure, or varieties of pigmentation or discolouration.

— The existence of circulatory problems, which range from permanent congestion to ischaemic phenomena. One must, in particular, take account of obstructive scar bands, in order to avoid the risk of necrosis.

— Alteration of the nasal valve can be demonstrated by the improvement achieved by lateral traction on the cheek.

c. Rhinoscopy should look for:

— A septal deviation, anterior or posterior.

— A perforation of the septum, a vestibular stenosis with adhesions or synechia.

— The location of the mucosal incisions, and the resistance or suppleness of scars.

— At the level of the nasal valve, the existence of an adhesion, the closure of the angle of the upper lateral cartilage with the septum, due to a deviation of the septum or to the collapse of the triangular cartilage against the septum.

Palpation of the mucosa using a cotton tip applicator, or transillumination can make it possible to determine whether or not a septal resection has been carried out.

Provided with all this information, the surgeon can try to reconstruct the scenario of the first operation in order to attempt to correct it, that is, schematically to:

— Complete inadequate resections
— Add cartilage or bone in case of excessive resection.

This new operation has to be carried out in a different spirit and the patient should be warned of greater difficulties with 'unpredictable' factors, which increase with the number of operations.

GENERAL PRINCIPLES OF TREATMENT

a. *Local anaesthesia* is used when one is dealing with minimal defects such as a projection of the bridge or a small depression; these are often minor retouches.

General anaesthesia is preferred in most other cases, permitting a greater operative comfort in sometimes long and difficult operations.

b. *The direct approach* through a marginal incision is preferable to see and correct defects of the cartilages. However, in the absence of defects of the tip, one can use a low, intracartilaginous incision which is often an easier approach. This is made below the previous incisions, which facilitates excision of the scar tissue.

The Rethi incision finds excellent indications in certain very difficult rhinoplasties, and the cutaneous columellar scar is practically invisible (Fig. 4.10).

The undermining often needs to be extended, because of the loss of suppleness and elasticity, and surgical manoeuvres need to be prudent; one must work carefully and gently because the tissues are more fragile, the planes of dissection modified by the first operation, and a tear in the skin or mucosa can easily occur.

c. *An extramucosal dissection* should be attempted if this is possible. If an extramucosal dissection has been done during the previous operation, the re-operation will be much easier; this is, however, rarely the case, but when it is, the bilateral septal undermining is extended to the triangular cartilages which are separated from the septum and the eventual resections carried out on the cartilaginous and bony structures; the scar tissue, when it is in excess, is resected with care

in the area of the mucosal roofs and, particularly, from the deep surfaces of the skin.

d. *The use of cartilage or bone grafts* requires a harvesting, and the donor area can be:

— The septum. When there has been no previous resection, a large quantity of cartilage and septal bone, vomer, and perpendicular plate of the ethmoid can be harvested.
— The auricular concha can also provide a large fragment of cartilage.
— Finally, the cortico-cancellous iliac graft may be used in cases where a larger quantity of graft is necessary, but the indications for this should remain rare.

e. *Length of time to wait before re-operation*:

— A discrete retouch, such as a small projection of the bridge, or an irregularity, can be done very soon (after the third month), under local anaesthesia, with a minimal undermining to allow the passage of a narrow rasp.
— All more important operations, on the other hand, require a delay of at least six months.

Among the sequelae of rhinoplasty, one should list:

— Firstly, noses operated on correctly from a technical viewpoint: the bridge is straight and symmetrical, the tip has no defects, but the nose is not in harmony with the rest of the face, or it is not accepted by the patient; this represents an error in judgement which could have been avoided by a better understanding of artistic rules and by a deeper psychological study of the patient.
— Secondly, noses which have defects:
• minimal defects which often appear secondarily, and which can occur with any surgeon, no matter how experienced,
• more important defects, representing 'ruined' noses.

We will deal with the sequelae of rhinoplasty according to a classification based upon the appearance of the patient in frontal view and in profile, the treatment of each being dealt with in turn. This classification enables us to list defects which, although they are discreet, appear more clearly in frontal view; the more important defects

Table 4.1   Secondary rhinoplasty

● Discrete defects: simple, rapid retouch, often under local anaesthesia
● Major defects: difficult operation under general anaesthesia

Detailed analysis
   History: — Previous septal resection?
               — Postoperative course: oedema, Polly-beak deformity?
               — Time of appearance:
                     ● Immediate: defects often major
                     ● Secondary: defects often more discreet

   Delay before re-operation: 6 to 12 months

   Examination: — Skin +++: thickness, suppleness, adherences
                    — Rhinoscopy: septal resection?
                                    thick scars?
Anaesthesia
Graft: cartilage (septal, conchal) or bone, or composite graft
Difficulties: variable

---

are apparent both in frontal view and in profile, being more predominant in one or the other.

IN PROFILE

EXCESSIVE RESECTIONS

This can involve:

— The nasal bridge; osseous and cartilaginous
— The alar cartilages
— The antero-inferior edge of the septum.

1. In the area of the nasal bridge

At the level of the nasal bridge, one can see a *notch*, a small localised indentation, or a *saddle deformity* due to excessive resection, either cartilaginous or osteocartilaginous.

A saddle deformity may be defined as a curve in the shape of a saddle, which is to say a depression of varying depth and concavity located between two heights or promontories.

In the case of a nasal saddle deformity (Fig. 4.2):

— The superior profile is made up either of the projection of the nasal bones which form a false hump if one is dealing with a low cartilaginous saddle deformity, or of the prominence of the glabella if a total osteocartilaginous saddle deformity is involved.
— The inferior relief is made up by the high part of the tip of the nose.

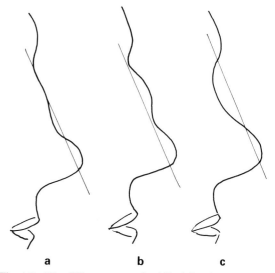

Fig. 4.2   The different types of saddle deformity. **a.** False hump with supra-apical saddle. **b.** Bony hump before resection. **c.** Excessive osteocartilaginous resection.

It is important to assess the degree of projection of the tip of the nose and particularly the ease of depression of the nasal tip when one pushes on it with a finger.

Among post-surgical sequelae, one encounters:

— The excessive resection of the cartilaginous or osteocartilaginous dorsum.
— The weakening of a cartilaginous fragment which is mobilised after reposition of the septum.

— The excessive resection of cartilage during resections of the septum where the surgeon has come too close to the anterior septal border.

The treatment of a saddle deformity consists of filling in the depression by various means:

— Either septal reposition
— Or insertion of material, that is grafts, preferably osseous or cartilaginous autografts.

a. The osseous nasal hump

The underlying osseous nasal hump adjacent to the saddle deformity is sometimes sufficiently large to be resected and used as a graft (Fig. 4.3).

This should be distinguished from a more discrete false hump, appearing after a previous procedure, which should be conserved.

b. The septum

The septum may permit a harvesting of a large amount of cartilage and bone, on the condition, however, that a previous operation has not created mucosal damage with adherences which make harvesting impossible (Fig. 4.4).

c. Auricular concha

Harvesting the auricular concha can be very valuable because of the ease with which this may be done, and because of the volume of cartilage which can be provided without changing the shape of the ear.

d. The corticol-cancellous iliac bone graft

This remains the last resort when all other donor areas are impossible to use or insufficient.

Several points in particular concerning bone grafts should be emphasised:

1. The tailoring of the graft is done in situ on the iliac crest, which makes it possible to more easily carry out the shaping of the graft with an osteotome.

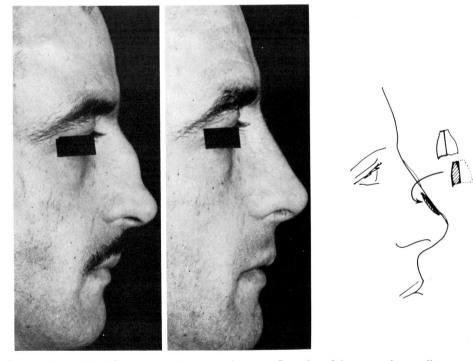

Fig. 4.3 Postoperative saddle deformity secondary to septal surgery. Resection of the osseous hump adjacent to the saddle deformity. Correction of the saddle deformity, utilisation of one half of the bony hump and of a superimposed fragment of septal cartilage.

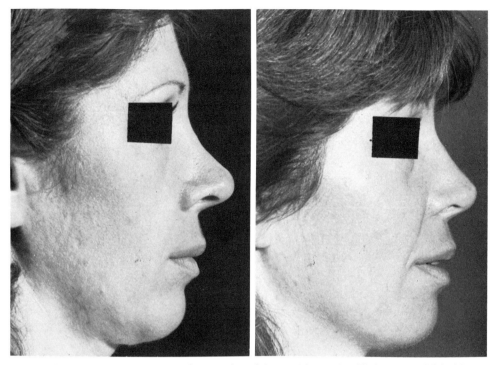

Fig. 4.4 Saddle deformity secondary to an excessive resection of the nasal hump. Equilibrium re-established between the receding bridge, which has been provided with projection by cartilage grafts, and the projecting nasal tip (lowering obtained by reduction of the lateral crura without section of the domes).

The bone graft should be harvested thicker than is required. Later, this thickness will be reduced in order to avoid fracture at the time of separation.

● *In profile* (Fig. 4.5), the graft should reproduce the curve of the osteocartilaginous profile line of a normal nose, that is, it should avoid filling in the naso-frontal angle and the region of the tip of the nose, if one wants to reproduce a normal bridge. The graft thus shows a convexity in its mid-portion and a slight concavity above and below (Fig. 4.6).

● *In frontal view*, the graft is thinned down inferiorly, has a small bulge in its mid-portion and then thins out again at its upper end. With this, one avoids the deformities often associated with bone grafts: projection of the naso-frontal angle, and projection of the supra-apical area with a thickening of the tip (Fig. 4.25).

The inferior end of the graft should not reach the alar domes, leaving a relative suppleness to the tip of the nose, except when a columellar strut is envisaged, or if a lengthening of the nose is indicated.

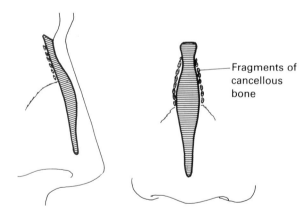

Fragments of cancellous bone

Fig. 4.5 Iliac bone graft:

2. *The bed of the graft:*

— The subperiosteal undermining should be sufficient to enable the graft to be introduced without force, and without creating excessive cutaneous tension.

— The wound is kept open in the nasal bones with a rasp.

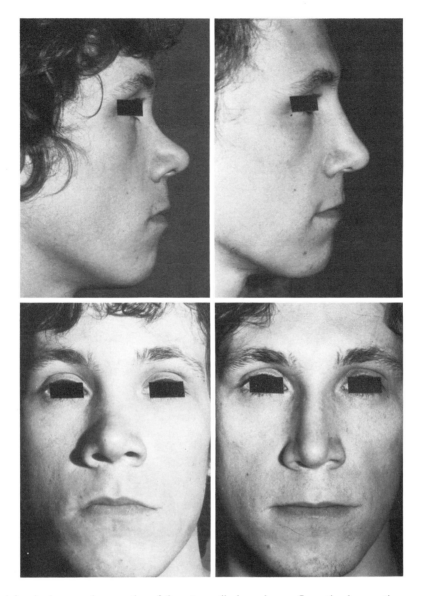

Fig. 4.6 Saddle deformity by excessive resection of the osteocartilaginous hump. Correction by a cortico-cancellous iliac bone graft without osteosynthesis or columellar strut. Lateral osteotomies. Note the increase in length of the nose that occurs with the correction of the concavity.

— A notch is made with a chisel in the upper portion of the nasal bones, cutting into the nasal spine of the frontal bone where the bevelled end of the graft will be placed. This permits one, in many cases, to dispense with an osteosynthesis. Fragments of cancellous bone can be placed under the lateral edges of the graft.

e. Cranial bone

The harvesting of cranial bone (outer layer of the parietal bone). This harvesting is not new and has been used particularly by neurosurgeons.

Under the influence of Paul Tessier, who first used cranial grafts in young children with Crouzon's disease or Teacher Collins syndrome, malformations which require operation in infancy, and large amounts of graft in the area of the face, the field of application has little by little been extended to the face and to aesthetic surgery.

There are considerable advantages to this harvesting: one can take from an operative field adjacent to the face, grafts which are of the desired size and contour; there is a very simple post-operative course since there is no pain or functional hindrance; and the scar is in the hair. Furthermore, this is membranous bone, where resorption is very moderate and where one can expect regeneration of bone after harvesting, thanks to a discrete local haematoma which forms over the bone.

Parietal bone constitutes the best area for harvesting, because of its slightly convex shape and also because of its thickness, which has been studied by J. Pensler and Joseph G. MacCarthy: this thickness is greatest in the posterior portion (average 7.72 mm, with a range of 4–12 mm). It varies with age, but particularly with weight, race and sex.

Technique:

— After infiltration, the incision in the scalp is made parallel to the sagittal suture and 3–4 cm from it, extending posteriorly from the vertical passing through the ear.
— The pericranium is incised at a distance from the zone of harvesting, so as to be able to later redrape it over this area.
— A bony channel of 4–5 mm is made by using a round burr around the area where the graft will be harvested. This bony channel should extend into the diploic bone.
— The outer border of this channel is burred down or resected with a chisel in order to obtain a plane of approach which is as tangential as possible so that the instrument can separate the graft from the inner surface.
— We prefer to start this cleavage using a very fine fissure burr and to complete the cleavage using a slightly bevelled 10–15 mm chisel. The bevel is placed on the deep side to prevent the instrument from passing through the inner surface.
— Once the fragment or fragments have been harvested, the edges of the donor defect are smoothed down and the diploic bone can be harvested with a curette or a chisel, furnishing large amounts of cancellous bone.
— Haemostasis is done with wax and one checks carefully to be sure that there are no breaches of the inner surface.

— The wound is closed with a drain coming out through a separate incision.
— This is a delicate procedure, not without risk, and one should approach harvesting a cranial bone graft with prudence.

f. Particular problems:

— The volume of the graft or grafts: if the local conditions are good (in particular, when there has been a good extramucosal dissection, permitting a hermetically-sealed pocket for the graft), resorption is minimal, or even non-existent; it is minimal as far as cartilage and cancellous bone are concerned, and greater when using a costal graft, for example, where cortical bone is predominant.
— The undermining depends on the volume of the graft and should be adapted to it so that the graft does not need to be forced into its pocket.
— Cartilage grafts can be fixed together by tying resorbable sutures around them. The widest and longest fragments are placed deep down, and the whole construction should be in the shape of a long, flat, dug-out canoe, thinned out at the ends, with bevelled edges and a smooth, rounded superficial surface.
— The construction is kept in place by catgut sutures which pass through the skin in the midline. This form of fixation, completed by a plaster or metal splint, is quite sufficient.
— Other, complementary procedures are often done:

• Reduction of the lateral crura
• Correction of a flattening of the nasal alae
• Projection of the tip of the nose by the addition of a columellar strut to the tip if the tip has collapsed
• Finally, lateral osteotomies should be done even with a bone graft if the width of the bony nasal bridge requires it. They constitute no threat to the taking of the bone graft.

2. A drop of the nasal tip (round nose)

This can be a defect when the nasal tip lies below the profile line. This therefore constitutes an indication:

— Either for reducing the profile line

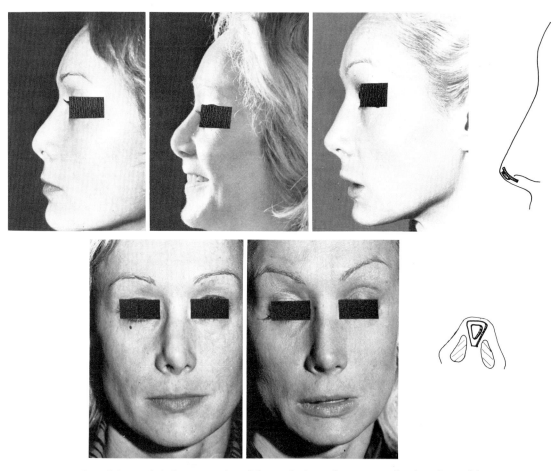

Fig. 4.7 Lowering of the nasal tip by amputation of the cartilaginous domes, extending into the mesial crura.

— Correction by: cartilage graft of the nasal tip (harvested from the auricular concha), using two superimposed fragments, one visor-shaped; moderate lowering of the cartilaginous bridge; lateral osteotomies.

— The fall of the tip is accentuated during laughter, with the characteristic appearance of a round nose.

— Or for projecting the nasal tip if the level of the bridge is in a correct position.

It is preferable, in these difficult cases, to begin with surgery of the tip, taking account of the width of the nose and the projection of the septal cartilaginous bridge. The drop of the nasal tip can be moderate, caused by resection of the domes with reduction of the height of the mesial crura which was not indicated. The result can be a round, non-projecting tip.

Sometimes, this drop can amount to an amputation with a very reduced nasal tip which is extremely unattractive (Fig. 4.7).

In these two cases, it is easy to make the differential diagnosis from a Polly-beak deformity, which can be associated with a retracted tip.

Treatment consists of replacing the missing or deficient cartilage with cup-shaped grafts, permitting projection of the nasal tip.

Several techniques may be used:

— The techniques described in the section on 'Grafts of the tip of the nose' each have their indications according to the extent of the reduction of the tip.

— The use of one or two superimposed cup-shaped grafts of cartilage, can be associated with a strut placed between the two mesial crura, which can be either a bone graft or a cartilage graft taken from the septum; this 'parasol' type of construction prevents the strut from rising up under the skin and makes it possible to give effective projection to the tip of the nose.

3. Excessive shortening by resection of the antero-inferior border of the septum (cartilage and mucosa)

This can be associated with an excessive resection of the hump; a saddle nose results, with a very turned up tip and nostrils which are very visible on frontal view. Treatment is often difficult; it consists of a lengthening of the nasal mucosa, osteocartilaginous support, and cutaneous lengthening (Fig. 4.19).

    a. Lengthening of the nasal mucosa cannot be done under good conditions unless an extramucosal dissection has been performed during the previous procedure. The difficulty is therefore variable, and increases according to the mucosa sacrificed during the preceding operations. One attempts, after an extramucosal dissection and an extensive bilateral septal dissection, to lengthen the mucosa by using a counter-incision under the osteocartilaginous vault, as we have done in the treatment of certain vestibular stenoses, where mucosa is provided by a high counter incision which provides a large advancement flap (Fig. 4.8).

    Cinelli's procedure can be used with benefit in patients who have a hanging columella. A small posterior septal flap is swung towards the anterior

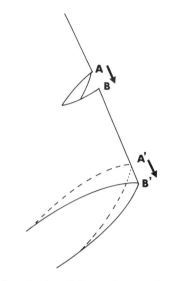

Fig. 4.8 Lengthening of the nasal mucosa by a counter-incision (A–B).

part of the inferior border, lengthening the tip and elevating at the same time the base of the columella. This procedure requires that the septum have a normal height or, even better, an increased height (Fig. 4.9).

    As for the walls themselves, lengthening is facilitated at this level by the reduction in the width of the nose after osteotomies. This mobilisation of the walls provides additional mucosa.

    b. Osteocartilaginous support is often indicated after this mucosal lengthening.

    Besides the bone graft with a columellar strut, sometimes necessary, the dorso-nasal cartilage

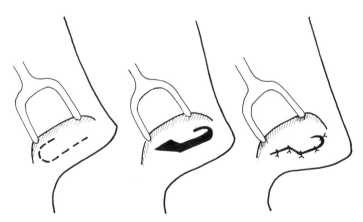

Fig. 4.9 Cinelli's procedure.

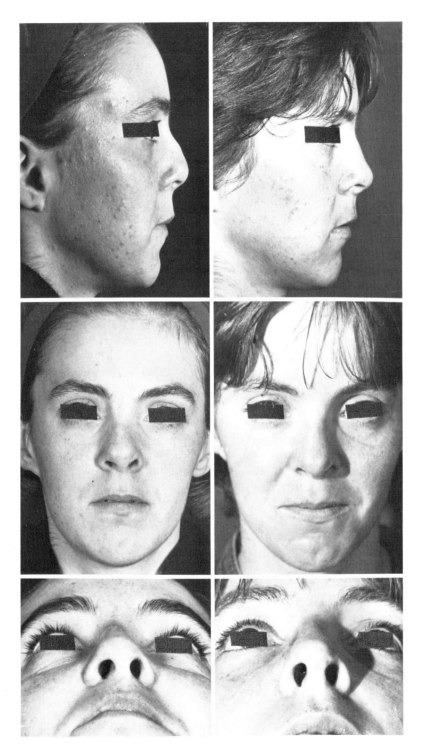

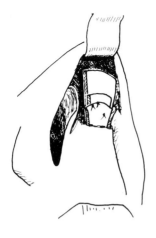

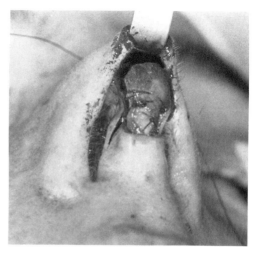

Fig. 4.10   Excessively shortened nose, amputation of the domes and the mesial crura.
— Harvesting of the entire auricular concha.
— Extramucosal dissection: harvesting of an osteocartilaginous septal graft.
— Tip: Rethi incision and cartilage graft of three fragments superimposed (sutured to the mesial crura).
— The bony hump is lightly rasped.
— Lateral osteotomies.
— Cartilage graft at the level of the antero-inferior portion of the septum (held in place by an X-ray film stint and packing).

graft is of great use because it gives the illusion of increasing the length of the nose by raising the naso-frontal concavity and by rotation of the tip of the nose inferiorly.

One could also use a columellar or sub-columellar graft (Fig. 4.10).

A graft placed under the columella has the disadvantage of widening it.

We sometimes use a procedure which involves increasing the vertical height of the anterior sep-tal border, by inserting a triangular fragment of cartilage (Fig. 4.11).

After performing a subperichondrial undermin-ing over a height of 15–20 mm the perichondrium is incised horizontally in its superior portion, then undermined in an inferior direction, this under-mining not reaching the inferior septal border.

A cartilaginous incision is made horizontally 5 mm above the antero-inferior septal border and the small tongue of cartilage thus formed is

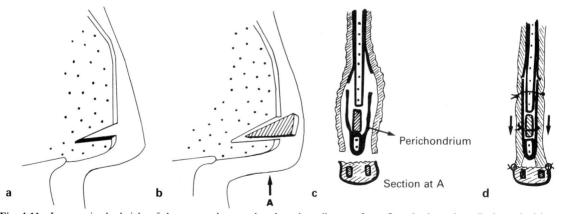

Fig. 4.11   Increase in the height of the septum by a wedge-shaped cartilage graft. a. Low horizontal cartilaginous incision. b. Insertion of the graft. c. The flaps, in continuity with the inferior border of the septum, are held in place by a transfixion suture. d. Transfixion suture above the graft.

lowered, pivoting on the nasal spine on which it solidly rests, thanks to the perichondrium which covers it on its lateral and inferior surfaces and which has not been undermined.

A small wedge-shaped cartilaginous graft is then fitted into the space thus created; its stability is assured:

— Firstly, by the greater thickness of the septum at this level
— Secondly, by a suture of the perichondrial flaps across the grafts.

The septal mucosa, after an extramucosal dissection or a counter incision, is pulled inferiorly and maintained by a transfixing suture through the septum.

Another, more simple procedure consists of increasing the septal height by a triangular graft placed between the two mesial crura and maintained by two or three transfixing sutures.

c. Cutaneous lengthening (Fig. 4.13) is possible in cases where the nose is large (because the mobilisation of the walls leads to a cutaneous excess), or where the skin is thin and free of scar tissue, or where the subcutaneous undermining has been greatly extended laterally and superiorly. A subperiosteal undermining by the vestibular buccal approach around the piriform orifice and up the nasal process of the maxilla to the infero-medial angle of the orbit makes it possible to liberate the nasal alae and the floor of the nasal fossae where one connects up with the undermining carried out on the septum. This lengthening depends in part on the reconstruction of the osteocartilaginous infrastructure. When the placement of the sutures has been done, a double hook maintains traction inferiorly thereby lengthening the nasal bridge while the dressing is placed (adhesive strips, then plaster); it is left in place for two weeks. The impression of lengthening can also be created by deepening the naso-labial angle, and by a discrete resection of the inferior surface of the nasal spine.

4. Retraction of the base of the columella

This constitutes a sequela associated with septal resection, and sometimes excessive mucosal resec-tion above the nasal spine which has often itself been totally resected.

The appearance is characteristic: the foot of the columella is retracted superiorly and posteriorly, and the columella is hidden by the nostril border. Here, there is a lack of mucosa and cartilage, and often septal adherences make it useless to try any mucosal lengthening such as the procedure of Converse ('sleeve procedure') and the Cinelli procedure.

Millard's procedure here has its ideal indication if the internal lining of the nasal alae (vestibular skin and alar cartilages) are present and of good quality (Fig. 4.12). It consists of transposing two chondro-mucosal alar flaps with a pedicle situated near the dome, into the intersepto-columellar space freed by an incision. Interrupted sutures are used; the two flaps are applied one to another by two loosely tied transfixion sutures and, in particular, by a packing.

5. Retraction-notch of the nasal ala:

• A localised notch in the anterior portion of the nostril border can be seen after a resection of the dome carried out too far outside. This is also favoured by a resection of vestibular skin, and a skin which is very thin.

• The elevation of the nostril border exposing the columella is associated with a significant reduction of the height of the lateral crus, and with an excessive resection of the lateral mucosa, during shortening. Correction can be made by reinforcing the nostril border with a fragment of the perpendicular plate of the ethmoid (the preferred material) and by the bringing in mucosa by an extramucosal dissection (Fig. 4.14).

IRREGULARITIES OF THE NASAL BRIDGE

These are caused by both excessive and insufficient resections. They are often not particularly visible and detected only by palpation.

Their treatment consists of a narrow undermining along the dorsum, making it possible either to rasp an irregularity, or to place a small, flat, thin cartilage graft, if irregularities persist in spite of the rasping, (a septal graft is preferred).

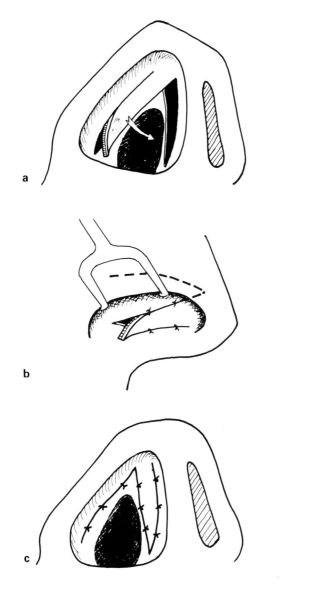

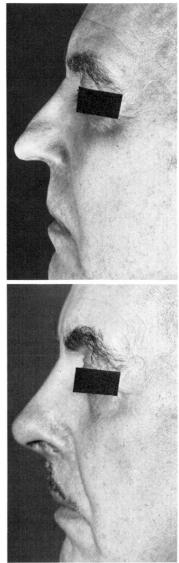

Fig. 4.12   Correction of retraction of the base of the columella. **a.** Horizontal columellar incision, extended anteriorly toward the dome. An alar strip (skin plus cartilage) with an anterior pedicle is taken from the vestibular surface of the nasal ala. **b.** and **c.** This strip pivots on its anterior extremity and this, on each side, comes to fill the free space created by the columellar incision.

This treatment can be carried out under local anaesthesia, and in a rapid fashion. The use of narrow instruments makes it possible to carry out the correction with very limited undermining.

INSUFFICIENT RESECTIONS

These are fairly frequent; they often involve the naso-frontal angle and the tip of the nose. Problems posed are of variable difficulty.

1. The naso-frontal angle

The naso-frontal angle can be filled in an unsightly way, particularly if there is a continuous line between a flat forehead without a glabellar projection

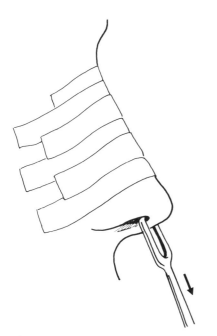

Fig. 4.13 Cutaneous lengthening.

and a straight or retroussée bridge. A deepening of the root of the nose is obtained:

— On the one hand, by a partial excision of excess soft tissue: subperiosteal dorso-nasal undermining changes its plane at the level of the root of the nose, and becomes subcutaneous. Working with the end of the periosteal elevation, one sections the periosteum laterally and superiorly, which makes it more easy to carry out an excision of the excess soft tissue;

— On the other hand, by reducing the osseous root by using a straight, bevelled osteotome, or a Mac Indoe chisel.

We should recall that the use of the osteotome with the shank guide makes possible a monobloc resection of the osteocartilaginous hump with the desired precision, notably in the case of a hypertrophic nasal root, and makes it possible to avoid these errors.

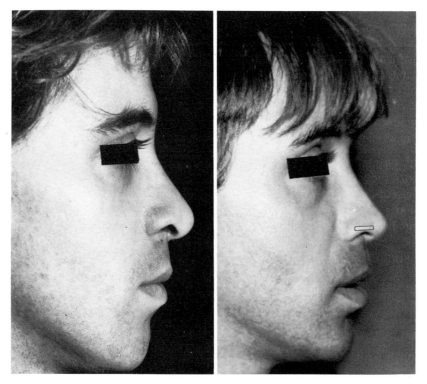

Fig. 4.14 Notch in the nasal ala: correction by mucosal undermining and insertion of a fragment of the perpendicular plate of the ethmoid.

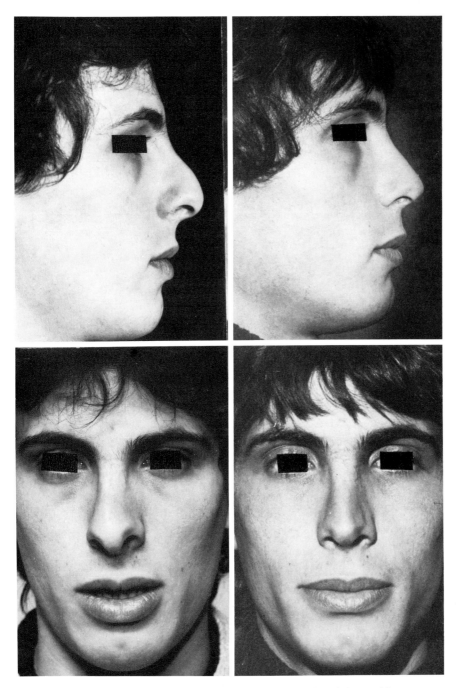

Fig. 4.15   Cartilaginous Poly-beak deformity, asymmetrical resection of the nasal hump.

— Deepening of the root of the nose.
— Lowering of the septal bridge and triangular cartilages.
— Reduction of the height of the lateral crura.
— Shortening and reduction of the nasal spine.
— Lateral osteotomy; correction of septal deviation.
— Alar reduction (3 mm).

2. The supra-apical region

The supra-apical region (located immediately above the cartilaginous domes) can present a projection, of varying prominence and unattractiveness, which requires operation. This is called a *Polly-beak deformity*. One may, normally after an operation particularly when there is thick skin, observe for several weeks or months a slight supra-apical hypertrophy. Massage, and the application of a cream of corticosteroid base (in very small quantities) can return everything to normal.

But sometimes, the supra-apical projection noted after surgery persists. Massage and the application of cream have no effect. One then speaks of the Polly-beak deformity (Fig. 4.15).

a. Several aetiologies can be encountered (Fig. 4.16):

• Inadequate reduction of the cartilaginous bridge and of the height of the lateral crura. The skin may be thick or thin; the diagnosis is easier in the latter case where one can sometimes see a subcutaneous cartilaginous projection.

• But the Polly-beak deformity can also be associated with a problem of skin of poor quality, and of the relationship between the cutaneous and mucosal surfaces — since the cutaneous surface has been preserved and is not retracted due to a lack of elasticity, whereas the mucosal lining and the osteocartilaginous skeleton have been reduced.

Thick skin should make the surgeon very wary, since a Polly-beak deformity can ensue:

— If the resection of the nasal hump has been excessive (there is inevitably a cutaneous excess)
— If the domes have been resected and the lateral crura overly reduced
— If the shortening has been excessive; this favours the formation of deep retracting scar tissue.

• Among other predisposing factors one can encounter:

— A short columella with a drop of the nasal tip during movements of facial expression; (recall the role of the depressor septi nasi muscle whose own action is accentuated by the displacement of the superior fibres of the orbicularis due to the action of the zygomatic muscles). This is very evident in the case of a nose with a hump and a hanging lip, and those of a short columella, where the tip of the nose falls during laughter
— A hanging columella
— The predisposing role of a transfixion incision extended to the nasal spine, which can involve a slight drop of the nasal tip
— A dead space between skin which is too thick to drape over a septum which has been overly lowered

The Polly-beak deformity, due to simple formation of scar tissue, should not occur if an extramucosal dissection has been done.

b. Prevention of the Polly-beak deformity requires that one begin with surgery of the nasal tip, if there is a predisposing anatomical factor:

— The extramucosal dissection makes it possible to reduce the extent of the endonasal scar tissue.
— A good adaptation of the supra-apical cutaneous cover to the underlying planes, without dead spaces, is important. It is certain that very thick skin adapts less well than a thin and elastic skin. In the case of a thick skin, the resections (resection of the hump, reduction of the septal bridge, resection of the lateral crura) should be limited and one can carry out a reinsertion both at the level of the dorsum as well as at the nasal tip.
— The resection of the depressor septi nasi. In cases of a hanging lip with a short columella, the resection of the DSN limits the drop of the tip during facial expression.
— The dressing should be properly modelled with adhesive strips over the supra-apical region; one

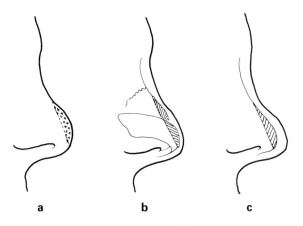

Fig. 4.16 Polly-beak deformity. **a.** Cutaneous excess. **b.** Inadequate resection of the lateral crura and the triangular cartilages. **c.** Insufficient lowering of the anterior septal border.

can also advise the patient to carry out for a month after the operation a nocturnal supra-apical compression, using a strip of elastic bandage 1 cm in width placed above the nasal tip.

 c. Treatment. Two schematic cases:

• *The skin is thin*, and the projection of the tip is correct: excision of the excess septal, triangular or alar cartilage is often sufficient to correct the deformity.

• *The skin is thick*, the bridge overly reduced and the tip inadequately projecting: besides resection of the excess cartilage, one must above all turn to reinsertions:

— of a cartilage graft over the nasal bridge
— cartilage graft permitting the projection of the tip.

The tip can be approached via:

— a marginal incision
— or a low, intracartilaginous incision; the latter makes it possible to leave a cartilaginous strip along the nostril borders, and to approach the scar tissue directly in a plane which makes it easier to thin out the supra-apical region. The excision of the scar tissue should be done with caution, since this alone is sometimes not adequate to correct the deformity.

In general, noses with thick, fatty skin, and with poorly defined contours, always pose greater problems. One can be led in certain cases (a skin which is very thick, or in excess) to carry out a dorso-nasal cutaneous excision.

A dermabrasion carried out above the tip can also prove useful in more discreet conditions.

FRONTAL VIEW

Frequently no defect is apparent in the profile, but the frontal appearance spoils a result which had seemed satisfactory — the result of the rhinoplasty should therefore be assessed both in profile and in frontal view.

Among the defects observed in frontal view, one encounters:

— Postoperative deviations
— Defects of the osteocartilaginous framework (dorsum and lateral walls)
— Defects of the tip.

POSTOPERATIVE DEVIATIONS

These are fairly frequent and can be:

 a. Known and pre-existing, but poorly treated. In this case, the deviation persists; it most often involves a deviation of the anterior septum, where the correction can require a lateral osteotomy and sometimes a graft of the dorsum or simply a latero-nasal graft if the deviation is discreet and the nasal bridge narrow.

 b. Pre-existing unknown, with discreet deviations which went unnoticed due to a rapid examination. They were unknown to the patient but do not remain so after the operation.

 c. As for deviations which appear secondarily:

• They can be *transitory*, and observed in the few weeks following the operation. Oedema more marked on one side, running along a lateral osteotomy line, gives the impression of a deviation of the opposite side. The examination of the nasal bridge seen from above when the observer is behind the patient, makes it possible to verify that the nasal bridge is straight and to reassure the patient.

• Also, there are the persistent deviations which are *discreet* or very discreet but amplified by the patient who dislikes his own natural asymmetry.

At the level of the osseous bridge, a discrete deviation can be treated by rasping laterally the osseous bridge on the deviated side, or by the inclusion of a cartilaginous or bony fragment to the opposite side.

It is necessary, if the result is good, to know when to abstain from being overly perfectionist, and to convince the patient of this. It is sometimes easier to correct an obvious deviation than one which is very discreet.

• A deviation of *moderate importance* can be associated with a high septal deviation which was previously unrecognised. The septum has a median anterior border, but immediately behind this there is an angulation where the bridge of the dihedron is more or less parallel to the bridge and near to it.

The reduction by resection of the osteocartilaginous hump therefore moves the anterior border of the septum laterally, and prevents the bony flaps, which have been mobilised by a lateral

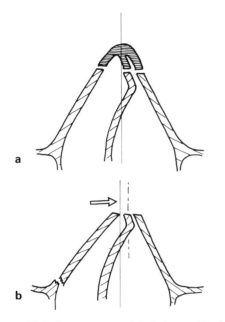

Fig. 4.17 High, inapparent septal deviation. **a**. The bridge is straight before the operation. **b**. Postoperative deviation (in the absence of correction of the anterior septal deviation).

osteotomy correctly carried out, to be placed in a symmetrical position (Fig. 4.17).

Treatment of these very anterior deviations is difficult. It can consist of a reposition of the bony septum after a fracture, or of a lowering of the anterior septal border; but one can also, in certain cases, turn to a cartilage graft placed over the dorsum or laterally.

Besides a septal deviation, the cause can be associated with:

— An asymmetric resection of the osteocartilaginous hump.
— Retraction of the partially resected internal lining, which can cause a cartilaginous curvature.
— The displacement of a bony flap immediately postoperatively: for example, an outward luxation with an enlargement of the osseous pyramid on one side. It is often possible, in the weeks following the operation, to carry out with strong pressure from the thumb a medial luxation of the bony flap (under pre-medication and local anaesthesia).
— If the bony flap has been overly luxated inwardly, an appositional graft (crushed cartilage or a fragment of the perpendicular plate of the ethmoid) is considered after six months.

Treatment of postoperative deviations is generally always more difficult, sometimes due to the mucosal damage previously created, but also due to the usual difficulties encountered in secondary rhinoplasties.

DEFECTS OF THE OSTEOCARTILAGINOUS FRAMEWORK

Defects seen at the level of the osteocartilaginous framework are most often associated with the lateral osteotomies;

— Either, the bony flaps have been incompletely or not at all brought together. There can result, at the level of the bridge, a hiatus (open roof), whose expression varies according to the thickness of the skin: a wide bridge, flatness or plateau, a lateroseptal groove, a 'break', or oblique groove.
— Or, on the contrary, the bringing together of the lateral walls has been excessive; this can lead to a pinched bridge.

1. The 'open roof'

This corresponds to a hiatus between the septum and the bony flap, which results from the absence of an osteotomy or an incomplete osteotomy, or from the absence of, or insufficient, resection of the osseous corners, limiting the coming together of the bony flaps. The extent of this hiatus depends in part on the initial width of the bridge, a very wide bridge being more difficult to narrow in spite of correctly performed osteotomies.

The appearance of the 'open roof' depends essentially on the thickness of the skin and the width of the bony bridge.

a. In the case of very thin skin, the 'open roof' can show vertical linear projections or depressions.

• *The median projection of the septum* is sometimes isolated, and more often associated with an insufficient lowering of the septum than with an 'open roof'.

The correction is simple and quick: under local anaesthesia, a limited undermining is performed, followed by a reduction of the septum using a narrow rasp.

• *A vertical groove* can also be seen between the septum and the bony flap. The under-surface of the skin is drawn into this gap between bone and septum.

When the groove is discreet, one can advise massage during the first few months with mobilisation of the skin to prevent too much adherence to the deep layers.

It is indispensable eventually to contemplate at least an undermining limited to the length of this groove, followed by the placement of a fragment of cartilage; a more extensive operation may be indicated if an evening out of the osseous borders, and an osteotomy seem necessary, or if there are other associated defects.

• The association of *three linear projections* (the septum and the two bony flaps) and the *two gaps* between them and the septum is the most characteristic sign of a wide bridge with an 'open roof' and which is covered by very thin skin.

b. In the case of more or less thick skin, one can note, according to the height of the nose, either a *heavy bridge* or a plateau-shaped bridge.

The *flatness or plateau* is seen in cases where the bridge remains wide and when the anterior septal border is not projecting or even when it is receding; one can then note the clear projection between the two anterior borders of the bony flaps defining a plateau of varying width.

— The preventative treatment should certainly have consisted of a complete osteotomy with resection of the osseous corners, and also of a cartilaginous re-insertion, because when the bridge is very wide, in spite of properly performed osteotomies, the bony roof will never close perfectly by the simple coming together of the bony flaps. In this zone of scar formation, the skin adheres to the nasal mucosa and one may see vasomotor difficulties associated with pain.

— The narrowing of the bridge can be obtained by:

• bringing together the bony flaps (low osteotomies, resection of the osseous corners),
• and by a cartilage graft placed as an onlay, which has an effective role in the thinning (Fig. 4.18).

c. A true 'break' is sometimes seen in the middle portion of the nose when the reduction of the osteocartilaginous bridge has been excessive in this portion, and when a lateral osteotomy has not been done.

— The appearance may be that of an almost horizontal depression, more often in an 'inverted

V' which seems to divide the nose into two different anatomic regions (Fig. 4.19).

— Treatment here aims to re-establish continuity, to 'establish a bridge' of some sort between the two zones, by the use of cartilage grafts (one or several grafts superimposed, depending on the case), the bringing together of the bony flaps by lateral osteotomies having already been done.

2. The oblique furrow:

This can be a manifestation of the 'open roof', but there are other causes predisposing to this condition which will be discussed later. A linear depression of varying extent extending along the junction of the nasal bone and triangular cartilage, the oblique furrow is most often bilateral, particularly when it is not marked, and thereby comprises the signature of the operation; but it can be also seen in un-operated subjects who have a broad bony bridge with a narrower cartilaginous pyramid.

a. Recall the anatomical connections of the triangular cartilages (see Fig. 4.20, and the chapter on Anatomy).

It is important to note that the lateral expansions of the anterior septal border constitute a thickening which extends slightly beyond the medial borders of the triangular cartilages.

The solid attachment of the triangular cartilages to the septum and the septal 'T' contribute to the support of the medial third of the nasal pyramid.

b. After rhinoplasty (reduction of the nasal bridge and osteotomies correctly carried out), the septal 'T' disappears, the new anterior septal border is thereby thinner, and the anterior borders of the triangular cartilages come together better along the midline; they *lean against* the septum and form the angle of an *acute dihedron*. The lowering of the mucosal roof favours this close contact between the triangular cartilage and the septum, and, in narrow noses, justifies suture of the domes over the septum in order to keep them apart (Fig. 4.21a).

The support of the middle third of the nasal pyramid which was provided by the junction between the septum and the triangular cartilage, that is, by the septal 'T', will be weakened because the triangular cartilages are sometimes weakened in the area of the superior bony insertion and no

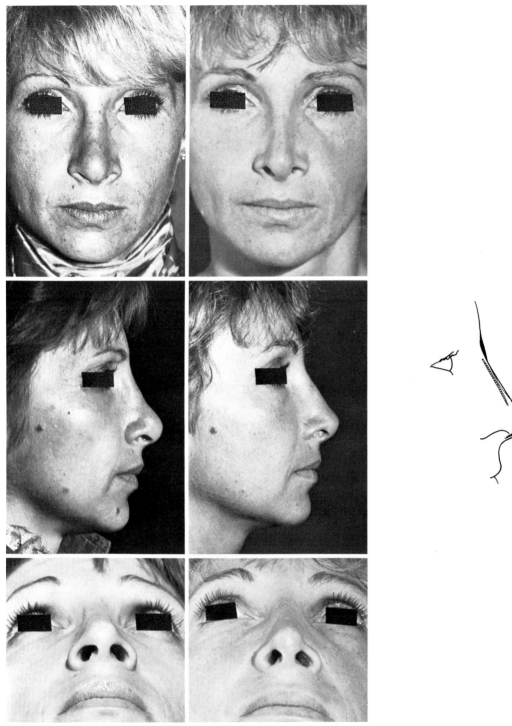

Fig. 4.18 Wide bridge (absence of osteotomy), naso-frontal angle inadequately hollowed, tip not reduced.

— Freshening of the naso-frontal angle (using a bevelled chisel).
— Reduction of the height of the lateral crura.
— Lateral osteotomies.
— Cartilage grafts: bridge (septal graft); tip (triangular graft).
— Reduction of the alae (3 mm).

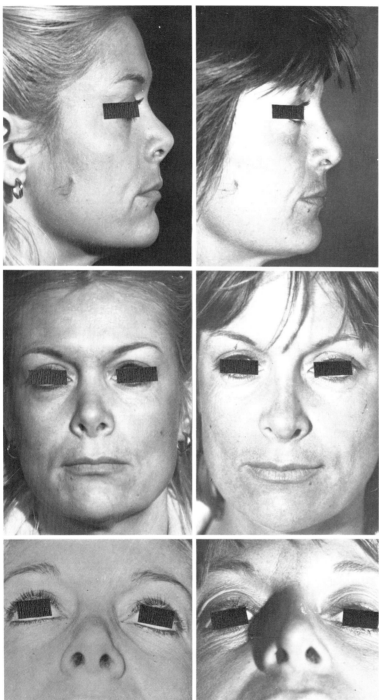

Fig. 4.19 Excessive shortening after reduction of the osteocartilaginous hump and absence of lateral osteotomies.

— Extramucosal dissection permitting a septal lengthening thanks to a high mucosal incision and cartilage grafts.
— Cartilage grafts (harvested from the septum) placed: over the nasal bridge (superimposed fragments); on the inferior septal border; at the level of the nasal tip (two thicknesses).
— Lateral osteotomies.

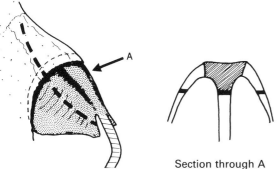

Section through A

Fig. 4.20 Section through (A), showing the thickening of the anterior septal border

longer have their solid attachment to the septum. Only the septal bridge therefore continues to provide the support of the middle third of the nasal pyramid.

The anterior border of the bony flaps approaches the midline, but not as easily as does the triangular cartilage (Fig. 4.21b):

— Because the anterior septal border is sometimes thicker superiorly

— Because the medial luxation of the nasal bone is sometimes insufficient

— Because a marked osseous curve, a very thick nasal bone and insufficiently resected osseous 'corners' can also be factors which interfere with this narrowing.

The nasal bone and the triangular cartilage which form the *osteocartilaginous flap*, joined anatomically, have at the level of their junction a separation which can turn into an oblique furrow.

This separation is further favoured by the superior disinsertion of the triangular cartilages during brusque manoeuvres of the rasp for example, and also by the reduction of the length of this insertion because of reduction of the nasal bridge (laterally, the overlapping of the triangular cartilages is less important than in the medial and paramedian areas).

The oblique furrow may be a manifestation of an open roof, but there are also other predisposing causes:

— Thin skin
— Destruction of the transverse muscles
— A significant resection of the triangular cartilages either by shortening, or by reduction of the anterior border.

*c. **Time of appearance**.* It is important to consider the time of appearance of the oblique furrow.

An early appearance, in the first or second month, that is, after resorption of the oedema, is often associated with an obvious defect which is not isolated: the osseous pyramid can be enlarged and asymmetric (Fig. 4.22).

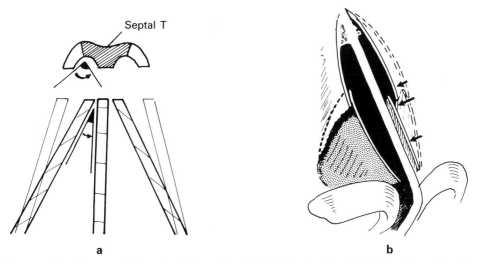

Septal T

a   b

Fig. 4.21 Factors predisposing to an 'oblique furrow'. **a.** Excessive bringing together of the triangular cartilages towards the septum. **b.** Accompanied by a disinsertion of the superior osseous attachments, and associated with an insufficient medial luxation of the bony flap.

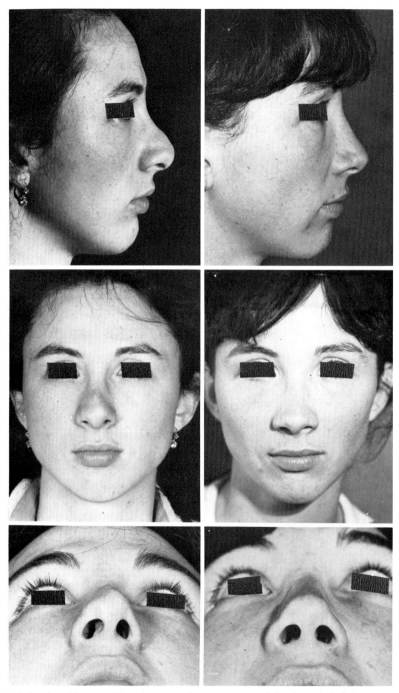

Fig. 4.22 Polly-beak deformity. Absence of lateral osteotomies, asymmetry of the tip and deviation.

— Extramucosal dissection.
— Tip: reduction of the lateral crura without section of the domes.
— Correction of a septal deviation.
— Bridge: lowering of the cartilaginous bridge and a graft of two fragments of septal cartilage; the cartilage graft is pressed against the left lateral surface of the bridge.
— Lateral osteotomies.

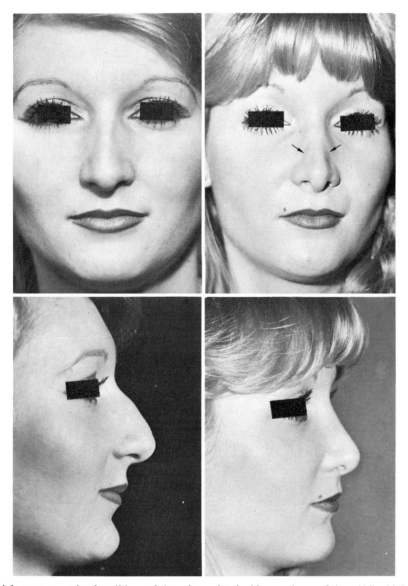

Fig. 4.23 'Oblique' furrows appearing late (14 months), and associated with a weakness of the middle third of the nasal pyramid, and the existence of very short nasal bones.

A late appearance, one or several years after the operation, can be explained by the disappearance of scar tissue (Fig. 4.23). Immediately after the operation, the bone and the triangular cartilage seem to be in a correct position. However, after removal of the splint, a discrete bony enlargement can be observed. After resorption of the oedema, the bone remains in the same position because of a solid, fibrous callus, while the anterior borders of the triangular cartilages move slightly and very gradually towards one another in the midline as the scar tissue is resorbed, associated with a degree of cutaneous atrophy. Thus, a slow and discrete medial translation of the cartilage takes place, relative to the bone, which remains fixed creating a hiatus in the osteocartilaginous flap which manifests itself as an oblique furrow.

d. Is it possible to prevent the appearance of an oblique furrow?

1. *Before the operation*: one can encounter predisposing circumstances:

• A rough outline of an oblique furrow can be observed before any operation in patients whose broad osseous pyramid with nasal bones projecting forward, contrasts with the narrowness of the cartilaginous pyramid. This narrowing of the middle third of the nasal pyramid may be associated with very short nasal bones, which, after reduction of the nasal bridge, causes the full weight of support to rest on the triangular cartilages, which have already lost their solid septal connections.

• The skin can also play an important role here; very thin skin being a predisposing factor, whereas thick skin always tends to hide contours and mask imperfections.

• Finally, the weakness of the cartilages, from the fact of their thinness, is also a predisposing factor.

The main prevention of an oblique furrow is by a cartilaginous re-inclusion along the dorsum.

2. *During the operation*: one should avoid rasping the junction of the bone and triangular cartilage with too much force, as this predisposes to disinsertion and tears.

• Avoid beginning the lateral osteotomy too high, as this weakens the insertions of the triangular cartilage on the bony flap.

• Do not undermine the dorsal nasal skin any more than is necessary, particularly when the desired shortening is minor.

• One *should*, on the other hand, *use* cartilage grafts without hesitation. The aim of the re-insertion is to reconstitute the septal 'T', that is, an anatomy close to normal. The graft, which is wider than the septum, prevents the excessive coming together of the triangular cartilages against the septum, particularly in their upper portion.

• The suture of the domes performed a bit high, can play a preventative role, permitting at the same time a better seating of the graft.

e. Treatment consists of placing cartilage grafts along the bridge (Fig. 4.24):
— Either a cartilage strip, preferably as an *inlay* between the anterior borders of the triangular cartilages
— Or a fragment of alar cartilage or of crushed cartilage placed between the septal mucosa and the triangular cartilage at the osteocartilaginous junction and a little below this, or else over the lateral surface of the triangular cartilage.

If the defect is isolated and minor, it often bothers the surgeon more than the patient. The correction can always be done by inclusion of crushed cartilage fragments after a narrow subcutaneous undermining along the depression.

The existence of other, associated defects requires a complete re-operation where lateral osteotomies, and resection of the osseous corners, are completed by cartilage insertions.

The association with a pinching of the cartilaginous bridge is fairly frequent.

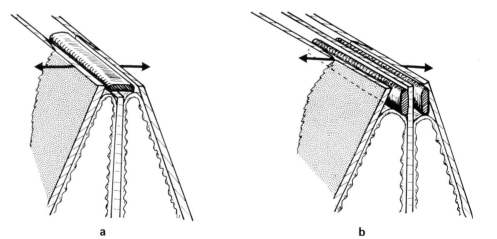

a   b

Fig. 4.24 Prevention and treatment of the 'oblique furrow'; interposition of cartilage grafts: **a.** As 'inlay'. **b.** On both sides of the anterior septal border.

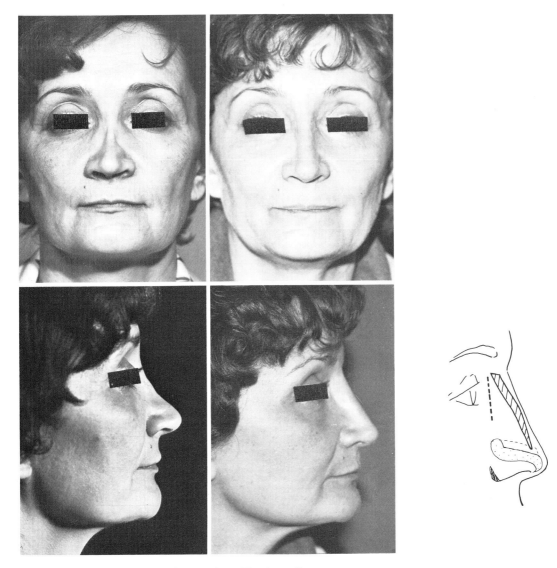

Fig. 4.25 Pinched bridge. Excessive resections. Flared nostrils.

— Cortico-cancellous iliac bone graft (because of the impossibility of harvesting from the septum), without an osteosynthesis.
— Triangular shortening.
— Reduction of the height of the lateral crura.
— Lateral osteotomies.
— Cutaneous resection of the alar bases (4 mm).

3. Pinched bridge — stair step deformity

Pinching of the nasal or cartilaginous bridge may be seen:

a. Early (Fig. 4.25):

— As a result of an anatomical or functional deficiency of the osteocartilaginous flap

— Accentuated by the juxtaposition of a thin skin to the mucosa.

The pinching can be associated:
- *At the bony level* (Fig. 4.26a):

— With a lateral osteotomy which is too anterior, with a stair step deformity seen at the edge of the

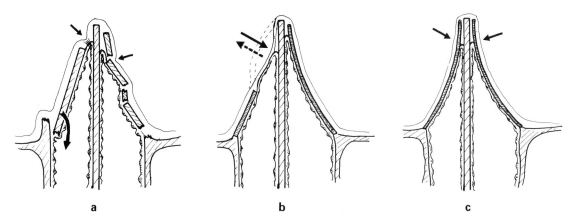

Fig. 4.26   Mechanisms leading to a pinched bridge. **a.** Comminuting fracture and lateral osteotomy too high. **b.** Subtotal excision of the triangular cartilages. **c.** 'Weakness' of the triangular cartilages.

osteotomy line, predisposed to by a tear of the mucosa during the lateral osteotomy
— With a comminuted fracture (excessive subperiosteal undermining also constitutes a predisposing factor)
— With a partial pulling-up of the nasal bone, in which case the skin comes to lie closely against the septum
— With an exaggerated resection of the osseous corners encroaching on the superior portion of the nasal bones, a thicker part which assures the stability of the osseous flap.

• *At the level of the triangular cartilages* (Fig. 4.26b and c):

— With a total or partial excision aimed at thinning
— Where the loss of all support can cause a thin and weak cartilage to fall against the septum, with inspiratory collapse and expiratory expansion.
— The other important factor is the existence of short bones. This fact has been well emphasized by Sheen: the presence of a largely cartilaginous hump with a short nasal bone manifests itself as a narrowing of the middle third of the nasal pyramid, which is visible if the skin is thin, and palpable if the skin is thick.
It is preferable in this case:

— Not to carry out a lateral osteotomy;
— And to reconstitute the dorsum with a cartilage graft.

In effect, after the osteotomy, the essentially cartilaginous lateral flaps lose the larger portion of their attachment:

— Cartilaginous (by resection of the septal 'T')
— Osseous, (even though there are minimal because the bones are short); the very mobile and reduced bony flap collapses against the septum, leading to a pinching of the bridge causing interference with inspiration.

However, the bones may have been overly reduced because of the reduction of the nasal bridge; the direction of the edges of the piriform orifices and its width then play a role: the wider the piriform orifices and the more horizontal the inferior border of the nasal bones the more this leads to create a drop after osteotomies and reduction of the nasal bridge, of a bony flap which is insufficiently wide to assure good stability.

b. The late appearance of pinching results from the same causes as the oblique furrow. Reduction of the mucosal domes is a predisposing factor.

The location of this late pinching is largely cartilaginous, the width of the fixed bony bridge contrasting with the thinness of the cartilaginous bridge.

c. Treatment consists in enlarging the pinched bridge:

— At the level of the bony flap; by apposition of two bony septal fragments (perpendicular plate of the ethmoid) placed superficially (Fig. 4.27a).

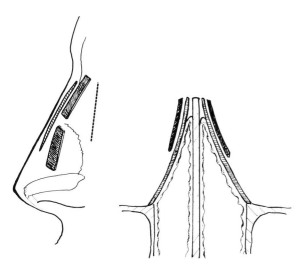

Fig. 4.27 Widening of a pinched bridge by thin bone grafts placed laterally and over the nasal bridge.

— At the level of the triangular cartilages: by placement over the superficial surface of the triangular cartilage of two fragments of cartilage whose purpose is also to reinforce this weakened, non-functional cartilage (Fig. 4.27a and b).

— An osteotomy which is too anterior should be redone using a thin narrow osteotome.

— It is often necessary to place a cartilage graft along the nasal bridge; in certain cases, where the pinching is associated with excessive resections, a bone graft is the only possibility (Fig. 4.25).

DEFECTS OF THE TIP

Given the variations and anomalies which can be shown by the alar cartilages, and also the difficulties in surgery of the nasal tip, it is not rare to encounter defects of varying seriousness in this area.

1. Asymmetry can be due to:

• A deviation of the inferior portion of the septum which has not been corrected, and pushes a lateral crus laterally. Correction involves:

— a transfixion incision
— undermining of the septal mucosa on one or both sides, followed by

— incisions or excisions of cartilage which permit repositioning of the deviated fragment.

• An asymmetric resection at the level of the lateral crura whose heights are unequal.

It is sufficient, after a low lateral incision, to undermine the vestibular mucosa beneath the incision, and to resect the cartilaginous excess.

2. A pinched tip

This is seen particularly when the skin is thin. It corresponds to:

• An accentuated concavity of the lateral crura which was not corrected.

A graft of two fragments of cartilage placed over the outer surface of the lateral crura provides correction. If the domes have come to be very close together, they can be separated by using a small cartilage graft (Fig. 4.28).

• A high section of the mesial crura on the dome, sometimes with a subtotal resection of the lateral crus or resection of the dome extending into the lateral crus.

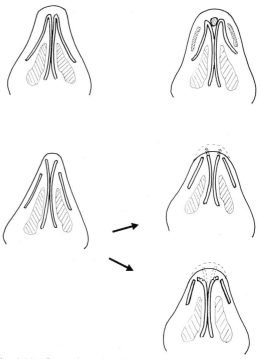

Fig. 4.28 Correction of a pinched tip.

If the projection of the tip permits, the resection of the extremity of the mesial crura can correct the deformity. One can also, by incisions on the anterior edge of the mesial crus, move the dome laterally.

When the lateral crus has been resected, it should be replaced by a small graft placed in the nasal ala. Here one uses preferentially a fragment of the perpendicular plate of the ethmoid or conchal cartilage.

3. Abnormal cartilaginous projections

These are sometimes associated with a pinching of the nasal tip.

They correspond to projections of the edges of the cartilage in patients having very thin skin. These are, most often, the anterior extremities of the mesial crura and the lateral crura, and can be associated with areas of pallor at pressure points.

It is useful, when a resection of the domes has been performed, to grasp the columella with toothed forceps, and push it up in such a way as to cause the cartilaginous extremities to project under the skin — one can thus more easily detect areas of irregularity.

Correction of a cartilaginous projection can be performed using a marginal approach. This consists of reducing and rounding off the edges of the cartilage.

4. Depressions and cutaneous irregularities

These are often associated with a defect of the cartilaginous support due to an excessive resection of the lateral crus which is in turn often associated with damage to, or an excessive resection of, the internal mucosal lining. Thin skin shows this defect more than does a thick skin and is more prone to nostril collapse on inspiration.

Treatment consists of placing a cartilage graft in such a way as to re-establish the support of the nasal ala. A short marginal incision, followed by an undermining which can be difficult, permits placement of this graft which can be either a bony fragment from the perpendicular plate of the ethmoid in, for example, a case where the support of the nasal ala has been broken.

5. Soft tips

These correspond to excessive resection of the domes and adjacent areas of the alar cartilages. The tip has lost all support, and it can be receding, relative to the nasal bridge. The excess skin can easily be pinched. The projection and the shape of the tip of the nose can be re-established in several different ways (see grafts of the nasal tip).

6. Endonasal adhesions

These can be either fine adhesions formed by the apposition of two smooth scar surfaces, or thick adhesions involving a large area.

— In the first case, a 'Z' plaster can bring improvement.
— In the case of a thick adhesion, correction can be carried out by 'minimal' excision of the scar tissue, followed by a lowering of the nasal mucosa by means of counter incisions located higher up (at the height of the triangular cartilages); an endonasal splint should be worn for several weeks.

In reality, this treatment is often very difficult, and one may need to use full-thickness skin grafts or composite grafts in certain cases of stenosis involving a portion of the nasal passage.

The sequelae of rhinoplasty are sometimes isolated, but they are frequently associated with one another, and in certain cases, fortunately rare, a total nasal reconstruction using an adjacent flap is necessary.

5. Case studies

1. DEVIATED NOSE

Nasal deviations can be cartilaginous or osteo-cartilaginous. They therefore involve a septal procedure which should be carried out at the *same operative session*; the approach to the rhinoplasty and the 'extramucosal' dissection facilitate this stage which can present a variety of difficulties.

Considerations

One should taken into account:

- The extent of the deviation.
- The osteocartilaginous or cartilaginous location of the deviation.
- Facial asymmetry and differences in the width of the two bony walls, and asymmetry of the nasal alae.
- The appearance on profile; hump or supra-apical notch.
- Previous septal operations.

Plan of operation

One should approach the rhinoplasty, no matter what the type of deviation, by:

- A transfixion incision carried down to the nasal spine.
- An extramucosal dissection; the undermining of the mucosa is carried out from the bridge to the nasal floor; it can be unilateral or bilateral, *total* or *partial*; it permits the correction of deviations.
- If there is an osteocartilaginous hump, it is preferable to resect it immediately after the extramucosal dissection; this permits a better exposure of the septal deformities, and facilitates their correction. Resection of the hump may be asymmetrical if the deviation is great. A 'monobloc' resection using an osteotome is always preferable, particularly if repositioning of the hump is considered (Fig. 3.6).
- If the bridge does not require reduction, a high section of the triangular cartilages is carried out at their junction with the septum. This is completed, after the lateral osteotomy, by a medial osteotomy which completely frees the osteocartilaginous flaps, and permits the completion of the treatment of the septal deviation.

- The actual treatment of the septal deviation is thus performed before the lateral osteotomies, and sometimes completed after them. It involves:
— Judicious cartilaginous incisions breaking the spring to permit the straightening and sagittal median 'reposition' of the septum, while at the same time preserving cartilaginous bridges to prevent septal weakening. One can use a spiral section (the 'Chinese serpent' of Jost), or a cruciform incision in cases of a curving deviation. In a case of angular deviation, it is useful to resect the top of the cartilaginous dihedron, and sometimes a strip of cartilage behind this bridge (Figs 5.1 and 5.2)
— The resection of an inferior cartilaginous excess is most often necessary: this frees the cartilaginous spring and is sometimes enough to correct a curving deviation by freeing the area necessary for replacing the septum in the midline.

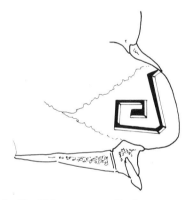

Fig. 5.1 The Chinese serpent (Jost).

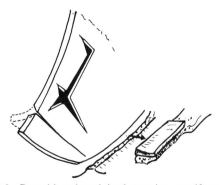

Fig. 5.2 Repositions by minimal resection, cruciform on the summit of the curve, and linear at a distance to 'free' and 'straighten'.

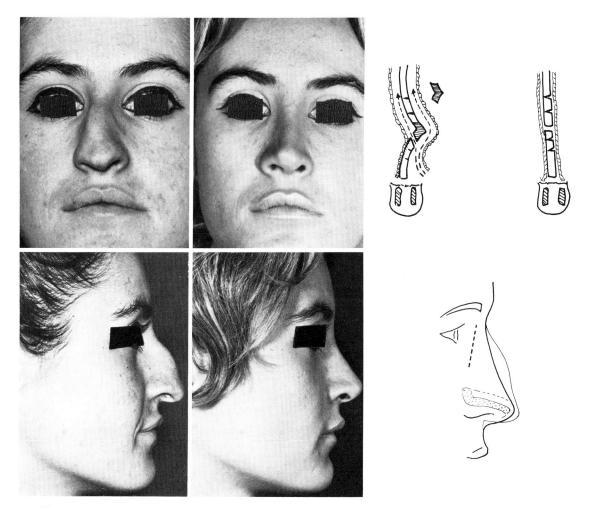

Fig. 5.3 Deviated nose with a nasal hump, columella slightly retracted.

— Triangular shortening (4–5 mm anteriorly).
— Resection of the osteocartilaginous hump with an osteotome.
— Correction of an angular septal deviation where the bridge of the dihedron is oblique:
  • Resection of a cartilaginous band at the level of the bridge of the cartilaginous dihedron, resection of the osseous and cartilaginous base
  • Alternated cartilaginous incisions
  • Septal reposition making it possible to lower the foot of the retracted columella.
— Lateral osteotomies and resection of the right osseous 'corner'.

• A lateral osteotomy is indispensable in cases of a high deviation. If the difference in the width of the bony flaps is significant, two osteotomies describing a triangle with a superior tip, create a zone of weakness on the larger side, facilitating the 'equilibration'.

• A splint to over-correct is indicated particularly in significant deviations (Figs 5.3, 5.4 and 5.5).

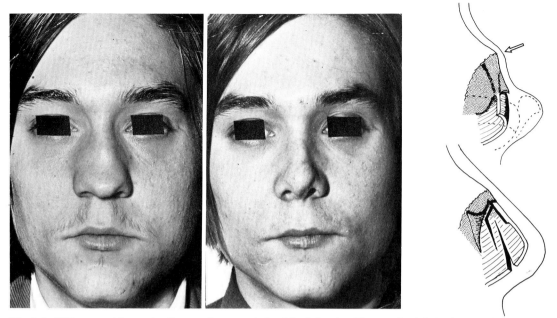

Fig. 5.4 Wide nose with septal collapse and supra-apical saddle deformity. The anterior-inferior border of the septum is folded back itself along a vertical axis, carrying with it the triangular cartilages and deforming the tip of the nose. The profile line is lowered above the nasal tip, with the formation of an adjacent false hump.

— Extramucosal dissection.
— Bilateral septal undermining.
— Section of the anterior border of the triangular cartilages, separating them from the septum.
— Septal repositioning by cartilaginous incisions.
— Reduction of the lateral crura without sectioning of the domes.
— Lateral osteotomies.

Fig. 5.5 Large osteocartilaginous hump with angular deviation and luxation of the septum into the left nostril. Soft tip.

— Extramucosal dissection.
— Reposition of the septum to the midline, by liberation and resection of the inferior border, resection of the base of the septum and cartilaginous incisions (parallel anteriorly and posteriorly).
— Tip: reduction of the superior excess of the lateral crura without sectioning the domes.
— Bridge: monobloc resection, slight asymmetrical, of the osteocartilaginous hump.
— Lateral osteotomies. The left median osteotomy makes possible luxation of the bony septum toward the right.
— Cartilage grafts:
  • To the tip: 'swallow-shaped' graft to which is added a fragment of the lateral crus
  • To the bridge: a fragment of septal cartilage.

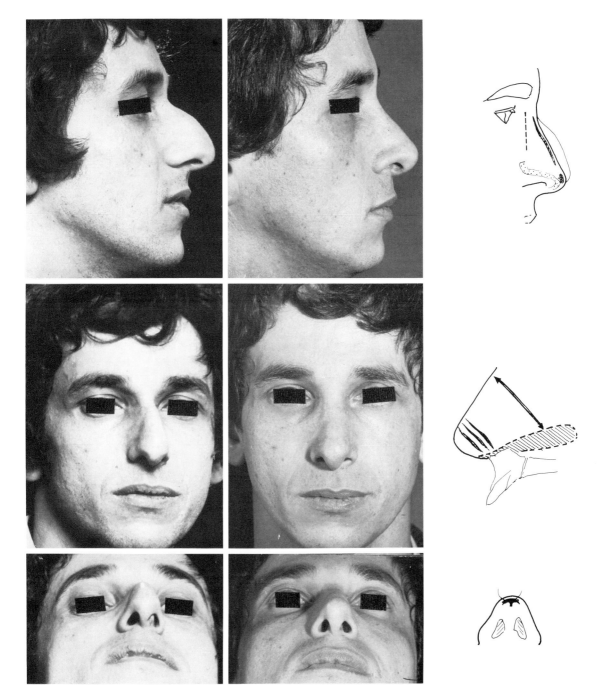

2. NASO-FRONTAL ANGLE (projecting root)

Considerations

One should take into account:

• The palpable hypertrophy of the soft tissues, sometimes with deep wrinkles between the eyebrows which accentuate the thickness of the tissues during facial expression. The retraction of the cutaneous cover after reduction is of little importance at the level of the nasal root, because the cutaneous surface is here less than over the bridge.

• The bony hypertrophy should be assessed in relation to the glabellar projection and the bony hump.

• The extent of projection of the ocular globes (the resection in the area of the root should be less if the eyes are projecting).

Plan of operation

• A resection of the excessive soft tissues (through an endonasal approach); the subperiosteal undermining at the level of the hump becomes subcutaneous at the level of the root; the end of the periosteal elevator sections the periosteum superiorly and laterally, facilitating excision of the soft tissues at the root of the nose.
• A resection of the bony hump extended into the root (by an osteotome or a bevelled chisel); a disarticulation is rarely indicated.
• A low lateral osteotomy with the resection of the 'osseous corners' if the bridge is wide.
• A re-insertion over the bridge of the re-tailored hump, whose upper end is thinned considerably.
• A compressive dressing using a metallic splint (in preference to plaster), which assures better compression over the nasal root (Figs 5.6 and 5.7; see also Figs 3.10 and 5.21).

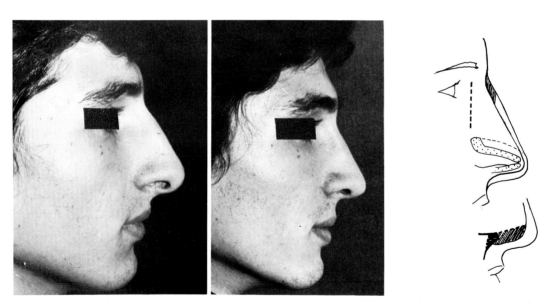

Fig. 5.6 Projecting root, nasal hump, short upper lip due to hypertrophy of the nasal spine and encroachment of the antero-inferior septal border.

— Resection of the hump extending into the root.
— Rectangular shortening (5 mm height) and resection of the nasal spine, permitting a noticeable lengthening of upper lip.

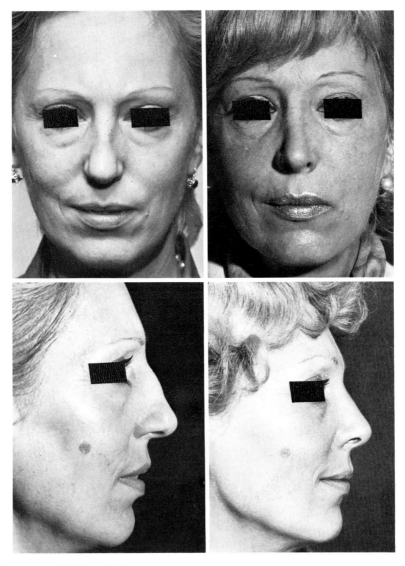

Fig. 5.7 Discreet hump, root slightly projecting.

— Extramucosal dissection.
— Triangular shortening (3 mm anteriorly).
— Resection of the osseous hump (osteotome) extending into the root.
— Tip: reduction of the lateral crura without section of the domes through a contralateral approach.
— Lateral osteotomies.

3. NASO-FRONTAL ANGLE (depressed root)

Considerations

One should take into account:

- The projection of the glabella
- The projection of the osseous nasal hump, accentuated by a long nose with falling tip.
- The varying degree of curvature of the naso-frontal depression.

A naso-frontal angle which is too hollow gives the impression of a greater volume of the glabella and of the osseous nasal hump; it is therefore contraindicated to overly diminish the nasal hump, which can appear even more predominant if the nose is long (and therefore requires shortening).

Plan of operation

- A shortening which, carried out initially, makes it possible to reduce the extent of the osseous kyphosis.
- A moderate resection, often discrete, of the bony hump using an osteotome.
- A narrow subperiosteal undermining in the area of the root.
- A reinsertion:
— In the case of the bony hump: a fragment of the resected hump or of cartilage (Fig. 5.8) can be placed in the area of the nasal root
— If there is no bony hump: one or several fragments of septal cartilage are placed over the nasal bridge, extending up to the root of the nose, where they are arranged in several layers at the level of the root (Fig. 5.26).

Fig. 5.8 Long nose with a hollow root and wide base. The length and the hollow appearance of the root give the illusion of a hump, which one must be careful not to overly resect.

— Triangular shortening (5 mm anteriorly).
— Tip: reduction of the lateral crura without section of the domes.
— Lowering of the cartilaginous bridge.
— Septal harvesting.
— Cartilage grafts:
  - Naso-frontal angle: two fragments of the lateral crura superimposed
  - Osseous bridge: a fragment of septal cartilage extending up to the nasal root
  - Naso-labial angle: a fragment of triangular cartilage placed in front of the nasal spine.
— Alae: 3 mm resection.

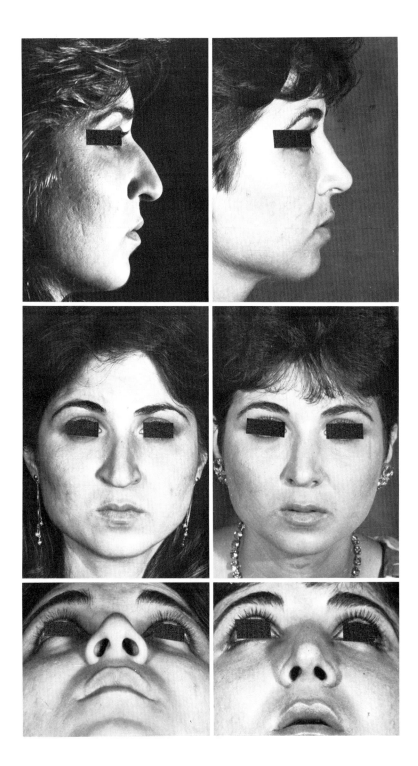

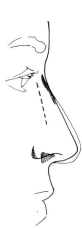

4. DISEQUILIBRIUM BETWEEN A RECEDING BRIDGE AND A PROJECTING TIP

This disequilibrium should be treated essentially by augmentation at the level of the bridge, which has the effect of reducing the hypertrophy of the tip which sometimes is not apparent or is mild.

Considerations

One should take into account:

- The overall appearance of the skin.
- The extent of the disequilibrium between the retracted appearance of the bridge and the hypertrophy of the nasal tip and its projection.

Plan of operation

- In the case of thin skin, it is possible to confine oneself to a reduction of the tip, but a better equilibrium is obtained by adding a small cartilage graft over the nasal bridge.
- In the case of thick skin, it is indispensable to 'advance' the bridge by one or several superimposed grafts; this makes it possible to carry out a less extensive reduction of the tip (Fig. 5.9; see also Figs 3.8 and 4.4).

Fig. 5.9 Disequilibrium between the hollow root, a receding bridge and wide base with hypertrophic tip.

— Extramucosal dissection.
— Tip: reduction of the lateral crura without section of the domes.
— Reduction of the septal bridge (4–5 mm).
— Septal harvesting and osteocartilaginous grafts:
  • At the level of the naso-frontal angle (rolled up fragments of the lateral crura).
  • At the level of the bridge: two superimposed thicknesses (cartilage and bone).
— Lateral osteotomies.
— Alae: resection of the base (4 mm).

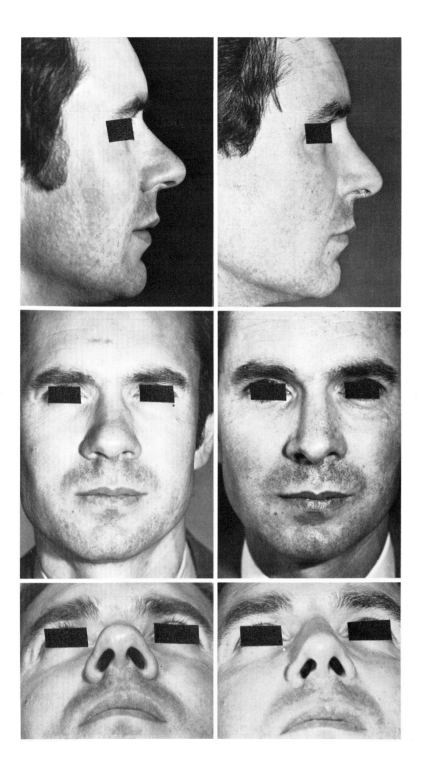

5. HYPERTROPHIC OSTEOCARTILAGINOUS HUMP

Considerations

One should take into account:

- The length of the nose.
- The projection of the tip, which determines the extent of the resection of the hump (the spring of the alar cartilages, the length of the columella, and the projection of the nasal spine).
- The width of the bridge.
- The width of the root.
- The thickness of the skin.

Plan of operation

- A more extended subperiosteal undermining.

- After an extramucosal dissection with a more extensive septal undermining, an excision of the bridge of the mucosal roofs if the retraction of these roofs is insufficient.
- A resection of the hump using an osteotome with a shank guide.
- An osteotomy with resection of the osseous corners in cases of a wide bridge and a projecting root.
- A reinsertion:
— At the level of the bridge (retailored hump)
— At the level of the tip: an augmentation of projection is indicated:
  - if the skin is thick
  - if the cartilages are weak
  - and if the columella is short, and if the projection of the nasal tip appears insufficient (Fig. 5.10; see also Figs 5.5 and 5.18).

Fig. 5.10   Large osteocartilaginous hump, hypertrophy of the nasal spine.

— Extramucosal dissection.
— Rectangular shortening (5 mm anteriorly), completed by a partial resection of the nasal spine.
— Tip: Reduction of the height of the lateral crura, without section of the domes.
— Resection of the hump with an osteotome.
— Lateral osteotomies.
— Cartilage grafts:
  - To the bridge
  - Columellar: a triangular fragment is placed through a marginal incision.

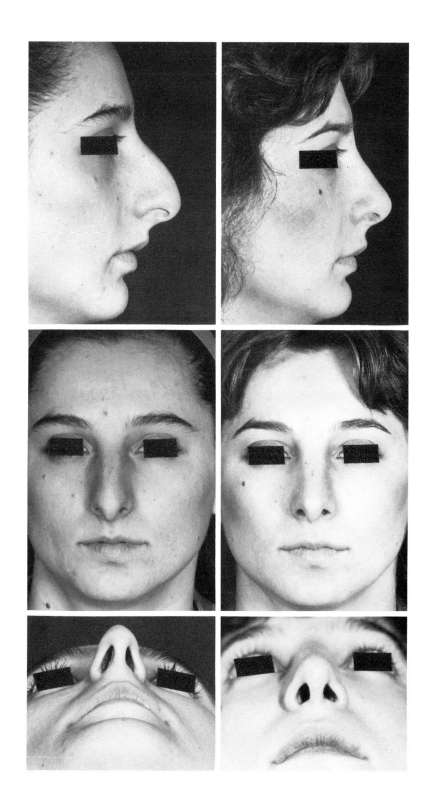

6. WIDE BRIDGE

Considerations

One should take into account:

- The thickness of the soft tissues
- The width of the root and the tip
- The curvature of the nasal bones
- The thickness of the septum and of the mucosal domes
- The presence or absence of a bony hump

Plan of operation

- A resection of the bony hump with a rasp if it is minimal, or with an osteotome if it is larger. The resection should take into account a possible reinsertion over the bridge, and should be followed by a reduction of the anterior septal border by 1–2 mm.
- A very low lateral osteotomy, followed by a medial luxation of the osteocartilaginous flaps permitting reduction of the nasal width. But this osteotomy should be total with a good mobilisation of the osteocartilaginous flaps. To avoid the risk of the nasal bones falling into the nasal fossae, one should conserve a periosteal attachment to the bony flap and should, therefore, carry out a very limited subperiosteal undermining over the osteocartilaginous flap.
- Resection of the 'osseous corners' and, if necessary, a thinning of the anterior border of the septal bridge, completed by:
  — A thinning at the level of the mucosal roofs whose thickness or extent can be a hindrance to the bringing together of the bony flaps. It is useful to undermine the septal mucosa by 1–2 mm to permit a slight drop of the thick mucosal roof.
  — A reinsertion, either of the retailored hump, or of a fragment of septal cartilage, is often indicated, particularly if the slightest gap persists between the septum and the bony flap, and also in older patients.
- In the absence of a hump, it is sometimes preferable to slightly lower the nasal bridge with a rasp, and then to place a cartilage graft (Fig. 5.11; see also Fig. 3.5).

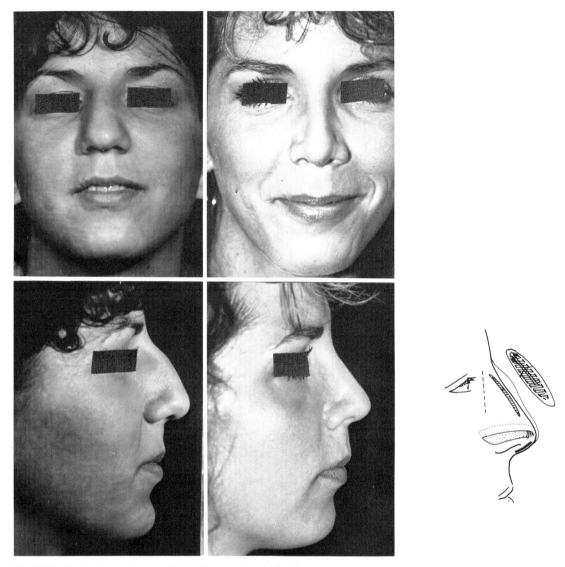

Fig. 5.11   Projecting nasal root, wide bridge and tip, thick skin.

— Subperiosteal, then subcutaneous undermining at the level of the root (the periosteal elevator sections the periosteum laterally and over the root so that soft tissue is removed with the nasal hump excised as a monobloc).
— Extramucosal dissection.
— Tip:
  • Resection of the superior excess of the lateral crura through a retrograde approach
  • Then a marginal incision permitting the exteriorisation of the domes, upon which parallel vertical incisions have been made.
— Monobloc resection of the osteocartilaginous hump.
— Lateral osteotomies and resection of the 'osseous corners'.
— Grafts:
  • To the bridge: using the retailored hump
  • To the tip: a fragment of septal cartilage is placed below the mesial crura, designed particularly to support the tip of the nose.

7. NARROW NOSE

A very narrow bridge may seem easy to treat. The skin is, in general, quite thin, and the tip moderately hypertrophic.

Nevertheless, after reduction of the osteocartilaginous bridge, one must check the degree of openness over the bridge and the absence of collapse of the upper lateral cartilages against the septum.

Considerations

One should take into account:

- The extent of the narrowing
- The size of the osteocartilaginous hump
- The appearance of the skin, often extremely thin, allowing one to notice the slightest defect
- The narrowness of the medial cartilaginous third.

Plan of operation

- On the bridge:
— a reduction of the osseous and cartilaginous bridge, usually without a lateral osteotomy (particularly if the reduction is minor). If a lateral osteotomy is performed, it should have an 'ascending curve', followed by an 'in-fracture';
— the placement of a cartilaginous onlay graft over the dorsum, the purpose of which is twofold: to fill in the 'open roof' if the reduction is major; and to separate the triangular cartilages from the midline. Keeping this graft in place is assured by a suture of the mucosal domes on which it rests, and by a suture encircling the graft and the anterior septal border.
- On the nasal tip, the skin is often very thin, and it is preferable:
— to conserve an adequate height of the lateral crus (more than 3 mm).
— not to resect the domes, or, if that must be done, to carry out the dissection very medially on the mesial crus (Fig. 5.12).

Fig. 5.12 Narrow nose, slightly falling tip, very thin skin.
— Extramucosal dissection.
— Tip:
  • Reduction of the height of the lateral crura (height of remaining cartilage: 4 mm)
  • Reduction of the tip by resection of the domes
  • Triangular resection along the inferior border of the mesial crura.
— Lowering of the bridge (rasp).
— No osteotomy.
— Insertion of a fragment of the lateral crus below the mesial crura in their posterior half: this makes it possible to obtain a better definition of the naso-labial angle, and better relationships of the inferior border of the nostril and the columella.

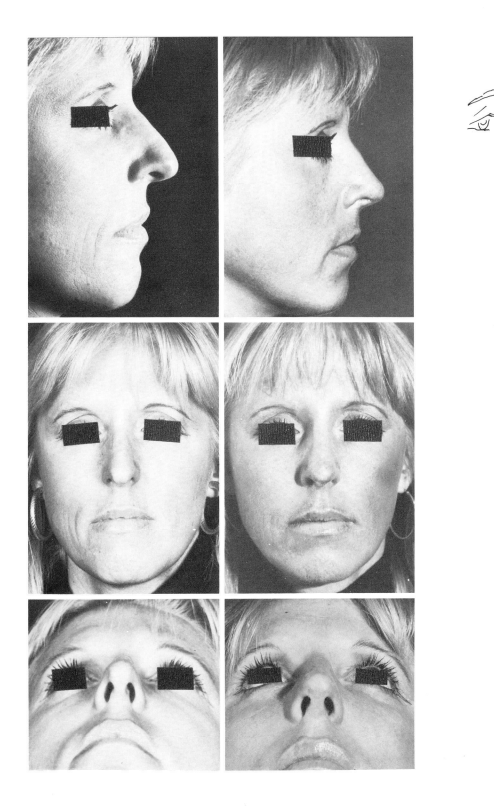

8. LONG NOSE

Considerations

One should take into account:

- The thickness of the skin. (thick skin equals less retraction.)
- The equilibrium between the nose, the upper lip and the chin.
- The relationships of the nostril border with the lower border of the columella.
- The importance of the kyphosis, which is less apparent after shortening.

- The location of the naso-frontal angle whose displacement by hollowing can give the impression of shortening.

Plan of operation

- An inter-septo-columellar incision extended towards the nasal spine
- A greater subperiosteal undermining
- Reduction of the superior excess of the lateral crura, and sometimes a section of the dome in cases of a falling and hypertrophic nasal tip
- Shortening (muco-cartilaginous resection of the lateral and medial pillars) (Fig. 5.13a and b).

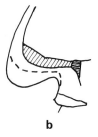

Fig. 5.13   a. Acute naso-labial angle with normal upper lip.

— Triangular shortening
— Insertion of the lower septal border between the two mesial crura with a transfixing suture (Figs. 5.14 and 5.14).

b. Acute naso-labial angle with short upper lip.

— Rectangular shortening
— Reduction of the inferior surface of the nasal spine.

Fig. 5.14   Long nose, hanging columella.

— Substantial shortening:
  - Rectangular on the cartilage (6 mm in height)
  - Triangular on the mucosa (4 mm anteriorly).
— Extensive subperiosteal undermining up to the root of the nose.
— Tip: resection of the domes and triangular, resection of the inferior border of the mesial crura.
— Moderate reduction of the osteocartilaginous bridge (hump harvested as a monobloc).
— Lateral osteotomy. Resection of the osseous 'corners'.
— Reinsertion over the bridge of a lateral fragment of the nasal hump.

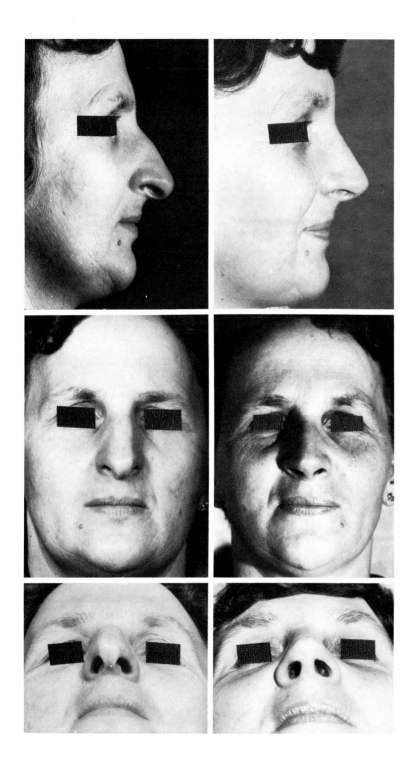

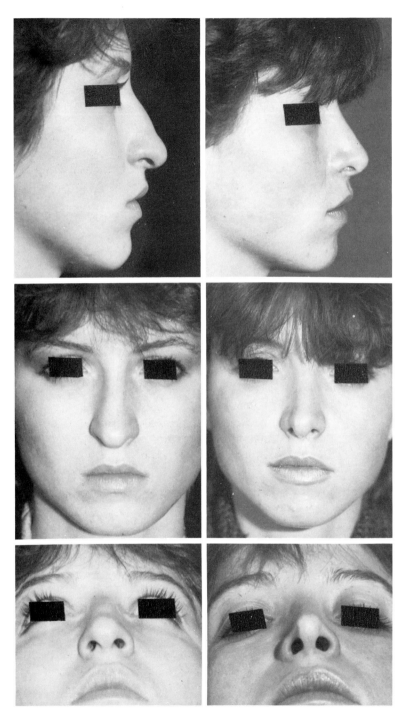

Fig. 5.15 Long nose, discreet hump, hypertrophic tip, discreet deviation.

— Extramucosal dissection.
— Triangular mucosal shortening (4 mm anteriorly).
— Rectangular cartilaginous shortening posteriorly, getting wider anteriorly.
— Tip: reduction of the height of the lateral crura (through a contralateral approach).
— Resection of the hump (osteotome).
— Lateral osteotomies. Resection of the osseous corners.

9. CLOSED NASO-LABIAL ANGLE

When the naso-labial angle is acute, one should consider the direction of the columella and that of the upper lip.

1. The columella can be oblique inferiorly and anteriorly in certain plunging noses, but it can be exposed in relation to the nostril borders.

2. In other cases, the columella is oblique but 'swallowed-up' to some extent due to previous septal surgery, an angular deviation or a post-traumatic overlapping of the septal cartilage. There is thus an elevation of the foot of the columella which is sometimes reversible by the correction of the septal deformity, which contributes to re-establishing the harmony between the lip and columella.

3. In other cases, it is the upper lip which has an obliquity more marked inferiorly and anteriorly; this is seen in certain ethnic groups and in certain deformities of dental occlusion. In the first case (a negroid or metisse nose), the alveolar inclination of the incisor teeth is increased, and a labial thickness which increases from above downward explains the closure of the nasal-labial angle. To this is often added a widening of the nasal alae. It is therefore in the upper portion, near the nasal spine, where one should operate to advance the high subcolumellar portion of the upper lip.

Considerations

One should take into account:
• The relationships of the nostril border with the inferior border of the columella
• The width of the foot of the columella
• The existence of a septal deviation and the sequelae of resections of the septum and nasal spine.
• The length of the nose.

Plan of operation

Treatment consists of:

First case

Triangular septal shortening (if this is indicated), with which can be associated a small cartilage graft placed at the foot of the columella (Fig. 5.16).

Second case

• Pinching of the foot of the columella with the effect of a projection of the foot of the columella; one often notes an elevation of the foot of the columella as well as an enlargement, the footplates of the mesial crura being placed on either side of the nasal spine (Fig. 5.17).

Correction consists of thinning the inferior septal border and the nasal spine along its lateral surfaces, then placing one or two transfixing non-resorbable sutures. A discreet, very anterior shortening can be associated.

Lateral osteotomies help bring the tissue toward the midline.

• Or a septal reposition if there exists a congenital or post-traumatic deformity.

• Or, in cases of a lack of mucosa and cartilage, use of various procedures aiming to provide mucosa and cartilage (see chapter on Secondary rhinoplasty).

Third case

The use of bone or cartilage grafts is often necessary, grafts aiming to lower the posterior portion of the foot of the columella or to project the upper portion of the upper lip.

One can choose between several procedures:

— Fixation by a buccal vestibular approach of a bone graft (the hump sectioned longitudinally, or fragments of the vomer) through the nasal spine with a wire osteosynthesis;

— Grafts placed in the area of the base of the nose as a modelling graft. These grafts can be placed in one or two layers in front of and around the nasal spine;

— it is sometimes sufficient to use a small fragment placed over in the area of the foot of the columella to obtain an appreciable change. It is easy to tailor a triangular fragment in the shape of an 'arrowhead' from the nasal hump or the osseous septal base (McKinney, Ortiz-Monasterio).

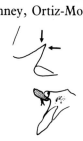

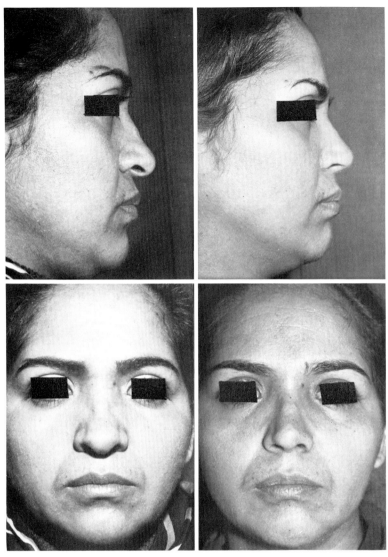

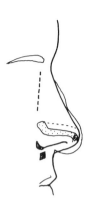

Fig. 5.16 Metisse-type nose, round tip, acute naso-labial angle.

— Extramucosal dissection.
— Triangular shortening (5 mm anteriorly).
— Tip: reduction of the lateral crura, staggered incisions on the domes.
— Bridge (rasp).
— Low lateral osteotomies.
— Cartilage grafts: two superimposed fragments in front of the nasal spine and at the level of the alar bases.
— Alae: resection of 4 mm.

Fig. 5.17 Nose with a large base, re-entrant naso-labial angle, ptotic nasal alae, supple skin.

— Extramucosal dissection.
— Tip: reduction of the lateral crura without section of the domes. Four mm of height of cartilage left.
— Lowering of the cartilaginous bridge (4–5 mm).
— Harvesting of septal cartilage.
— Insertion of two fragments of superimposed cartilage placed behind the base of the columella.
— Lateral osteotomies.
— Alae: resection of the alar base (4 mm); cutaneous resection along the inferior border of the nasal ala (Millard).

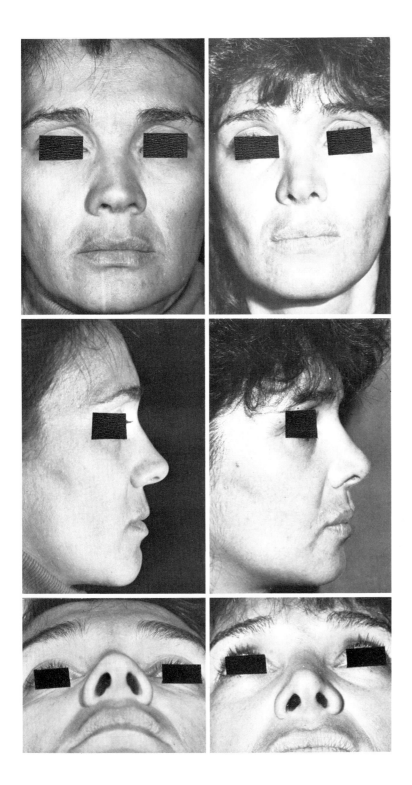

10. OPEN NASO-LABIAL ANGLE

Considerations

One should take into account:

- The height of the upper lip:
— if short, it permits the hollowing of the naso-labial angle and the lengthening of the upper lip
— if long, it requires a more modest hollowing and a slight lengthening of the nose
- The width of the foot of the columella whose pinching may oppose the hollowing of the naso-labial angle: often, this is due to an inferior septal border which is wide and luxated from the nasal spine
- The projection of the nasal tip
- The width of the nose
- The extent of projection of the nasal spine.

Plan of operation

- Prolong the intersepto-columellar incision to the nasal spine.
- Excise the tissues covering the nasal spine.
- Dissect subperiosteally the nasal spine on all of its surfaces.
- Resect the lateral borders and the inferior surface of the nasal spine using a rongeur.
- Excise the inferior septal border (to a height depending on the desired elevation).
- Place a cartilage graft of the nasal tip which may drop further after hollowing of the nasal spine.
- In the case of a short nose, a hollowing of the naso-labial angle may be associated with a dorso-nasal graft and a graft of the nasal tip (sub-columellar) (Fig. 5.18; see also Fig. 5.10 and 5.33).

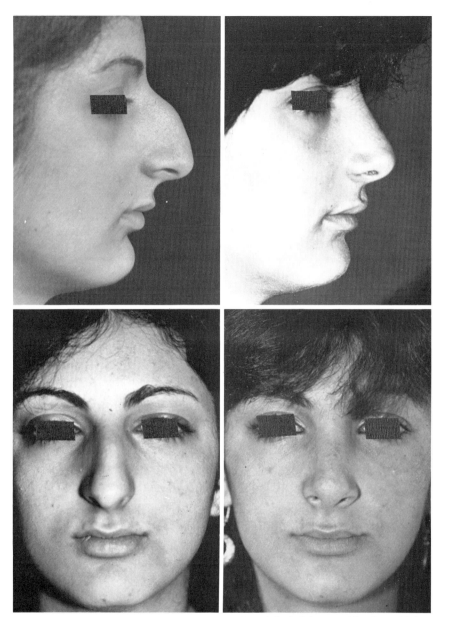

Fig. 5.18 Large osteocartilaginous hump, projection of the inferior septal border, with hypertrophy of the nasal spine. The projection of the nasal tip, which may appear satisfactory, will be insufficient after lowering of the cartilaginous bridge and reduction of the nasal spine, and will require a columellar graft.

— Extramucosal dissection.
— Shortening and resection of the very hypertrophic nasal spine.
— Reduction of the lateral crura without section of the domes.
— Lateral osteotomies; resection of the 'osseous corners'.
— Resection of the mucosal roofs extending on both sides of the septum and hindering the bringing together of the osteocartilaginous flaps.
— Grafts over the dorsum (cartilage fragment) and columella (osseous fragment taken from the hump).

11. HANGING COLUMELLA

Considerations

One should take into account:

- The height and the curve of the mesial crura
- The curve of the inferior septal border
- Whether or not the level of the nostril border is much raised.

Plan of operation

- A moderate resection of the superior excess of the lateral crura

- A resection of the inferior septal border (shortening of the mucosa and cartilage) (Fig. 5.14)
- An elliptical excision in the thickness of the columella, involving skin and cartilage, if the extent of hanging is significant.

The more the curvature of the inferior border is pronounced, the lower this excision should be (Fig. 5.19).

Also, the height of this excision should leave a normal height of the mesial crus.

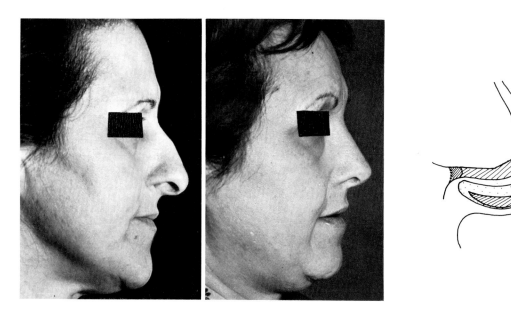

Fig. 5.19 Hanging columella, nasal hump.

— Septum: rectangular shortening with a double angle (height: 5–6 mm); partial resection of the nasal spine.
— Columella: fusiform horizontal resection in the inferior portion of the mesial crura.
— Alar cartilages, moderate reduction of the lateral crus without section of the domes.

12. ALAR COLLAPSE. WIDE BASE OF COLUMELLA

Certain patients complain of greater respiratory difficulty during inspiration: There is at this time a **collapse of the nasal ala** against the septum. When these abnormalities are observed during inspiration, one must seek the cause in the nasal vestibule.

Considerations

One should take into account:

- The length of the nose (falling tip).
- The narrowness of the nostril orifices.
- The broadening of the columella and of its base.
- A cartilaginous dome with an acute angle.
- The thickness of the septum and of the nasal spine.
- Soft nasal alae which are supported by soft cartilages.
- A narrow piriform aperture.

Plan of operation

- A septal correction if this is necessary.
- Reinforcing a weak lateral crus by using a fragment of cartilage (concha) or perpendicular plate of the ethmoid
- Not sectioning the domes
- Sometimes, the necessity of enlarging the piriform orifice through a buccal approach
- Fomon's procedure, which consists of passing the inferior borders of the upper lateral cartilages over the superficial surface of the lateral crura
- Reduction of the width of the base of the columella.

The width of the foot of the columella has several causes which should be studied in order to carry out proper treatment.

Considerations

One should take into account:

- The exaggerated curvature of the posterior extremities of the mesial crura
- The presence of excess soft tissue between the foot plates of the mesial crura
- The projection of the nasal spine
- The enlargement of the inferior septal border
- A frequent displacement of the inferior septal border to one side.

Plan of operation

- Excision of the hypertrophied foot plates of the medial crura, and sometimes a discreet resection of the septal mucosa, making it possible to 'return' the skin of the mesial footplate into the nostril.
- Excision of the soft tissues in the area of the foot of the columella between the foot plates of the mesial crura
- In particular, reduction of the lateral surfaces of the nasal spine (generally, more on one side than the other).
- Reduction of the inferior septal border which is alone sometimes sufficient to correct the deformity: it can be resected (shortened) or thinned.
- Suture by one or two non-resorbable sutures; this suture has the effect of slightly opening the naso-labial angle (transfixing sutures), by projecting the soft tissues (Figs 5.20 and 5.21).

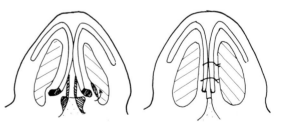

Fig. 5.20

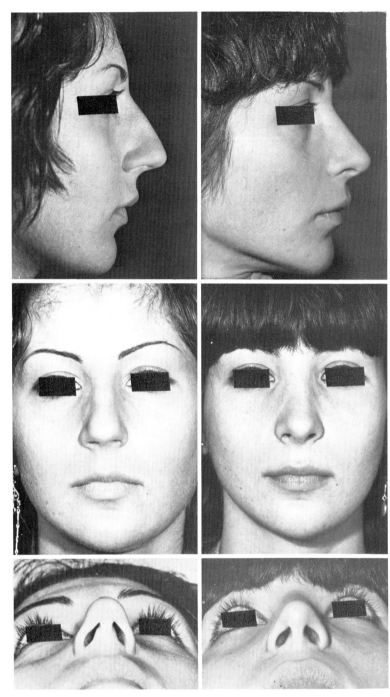

Fig. 5.21 Nasal hump, projecting root, wide base of columella.

— Triangular anterior mucosal shortening.
— Reduction of the lateral surfaces of the nasal spine.
— Thinning of the inferior septal border.
— Reduction of the height of the lateral crura without section of the domes.
— Excision of the foot plates of the mesial crura.
— Lateral osteotomies; resection of the osseous 'corners'.
— Suture of the base of the columella by two transfixing incisions (Non-resorbable suture).
— Alae: resection (3 mm).

13. THICK SKIN

The lack of definition, and the rounded aspect of the tip of the nose sometimes make hazardous a reduction, so that, when it is carried out it should always be moderate.

In fact, augmentation by grafts on the bridge and the nasal tip is desirable in certain cases.

Plan of operation

● A low intracartilaginous incision and a large in-filtration with anaesthetic, with the dissection carried out flush with the deep surface of the skin cover, which then permits the excision of all the tissues covering the alar and triangular cartilages.

● A low incision facilitates the surgery of the tip which is always more delicate when the skin is thick and lacking in suppleness.

● Nevertheless, it is necessary to conserve a height of cartilage of at least 4 mm, if the cartilage is thin and weak; this height can be reduced if one encounters a thick, firm cartilage.

● The shortening of a nose with thick skin can only be moderate, and in certain rare cases with very thick skin, an external cutaneous resection is indicated.

One can classify thick skins into two types:

— Skin of intermediate thickness, where reduction is possible but should be conservative (see Figs 5.22 and 5.23, pp. 154–155; see also Fig. 3.8)

— A very thick skin where it is necessary to:
  ● avoid all reduction
  ● prefer cartilage grafts over the bridge and, in particular, in the tip of the nose, by a rigid columellar strut resting on the nasal spine, associated with a conchal graft (in the case of a short columella)
  ● consider sometimes, a dorsal cutaneous excision, and often
  ● do nothing . . .

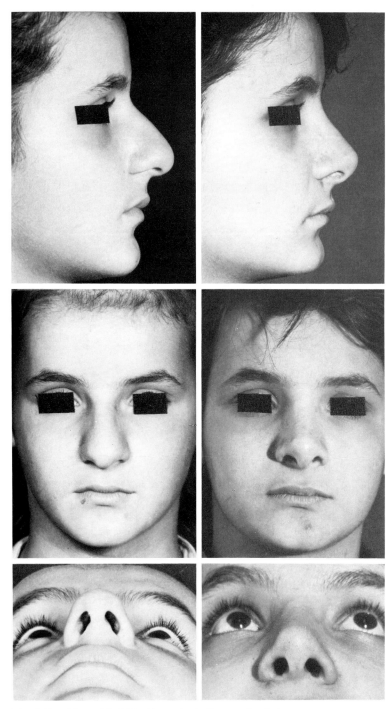

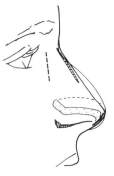

Fig. 5.22   Nose with thick skin, and a bulbous and soft tip.

— Extramucosal dissection.
— Tip: exteriorisation of the domes and reduction of the superior excess of the lateral crura.
— Triangular shortening (3 mm anteriorly).
— Insertion of a fragment of the lateral crus extending up to the root of the nose.
— Cartilage graft for support of the nasal tip (septal cartilage).
— Lateral osteotomies.
— Alae: 3 mm reduction and thinning of the nasal ala.

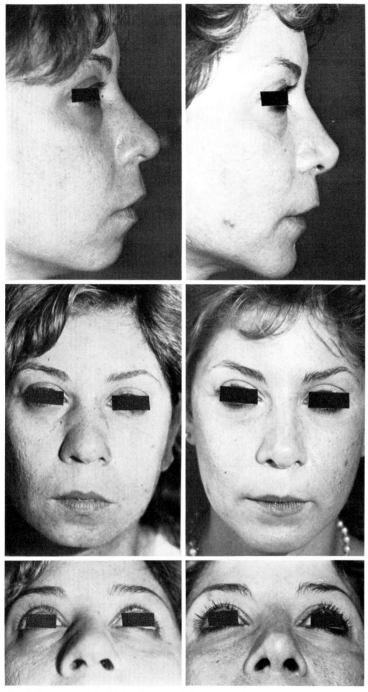

Fig. 5.23 Nose with thick skin, round tip, retrogenia.

— Osteotomy of the chin with 10 mm advancement (osteosynthesis with three wires).
— Nose:
- Extramucosal dissection
- Tip: retrograde undermining and reduction of the superior excess of the lateral crura, without section of the domes; marginal incision and exteriorisation of the domes upon which staggered incisions are carried out
- Harvesting of septal cartilage
- Lateral osteotomies and in-fracture
- Cartilage grafts: over the bridge (onlay graft); on the tip (Sheen's triangular graft); in front of the nasal spine;
- Alae: cutaneous resection (width 3 mm).

14. NEGROID NOSE

The problem is rather different for American blacks, for example, who live in the United States, and the blacks who work in France but preserve deep attachments to their own countries of origin where they wish to return. The respiratory problems are not the same in these African countries, particularly in hot and humid climates, as they are in France. It is not by chance that blacks have wide nostrils; it is an adaptation to the environment and we should not forget this.

The negroid nose is characterised by a broad, flat bridge, a broad base with a flattened alae and a marked alar groove; the naso-labial angle is acute and re-entrant, due in part to the marked obliquity of the upper lip which is sometimes significally thickened in its labial segment.

Anatomically: the nasal bones are often short, the piriform orifice enlarged, the triangular cartilages small and triangular, and the alar cartilages soft and without firmness. The septum is rarely deviated; its antero-superior border is receding and, rather than a retraction of the nasal bridge, it is a projection of the latter which one seeks during correction.

As for the antero-inferior border of the septum, it is also receding as compared to a caucasian nose; it is therefore rarely necessary to shorten the nose. The tip of the nose is flattened, with a short columella and nostril orifices with a greater transverse distance, the alae often being very flattened. A cartilage graft in front of the nasal spine is usually indispensable.

Plan of operation

In general, its operation involves (Fig. 5.24):

• Projection of the nasal bridge by a bone or cartilage graft
• A low lateral osteotomy, but the bones are short and there is a risk of their falling into the nasal fossae
• At the level of the nasal tip: a columellar strut resting on the nasal spine combined with a 'parasol-shaped' cartilage graft
• Resection of the foot on the nostril alae.

Fig. 5.24 Negroid nose, wide flattened tip, alae flared, low bridge.
— Extramucosal dissection.
— Tip: resection of the superior excess of the lateral crura, and staggered incisions over the domes.
— Septal harvesting and grafts:
   • On the tip: a triangular fragment under the columella; two fragments of the lateral crus (fleur-de-lys)
   • On the bridge: three superimposed fragments
   • Naso-labial angle: a fragment of lateral crus in a spiral.
— Cutaneous excision of the alar bases (3 mm).

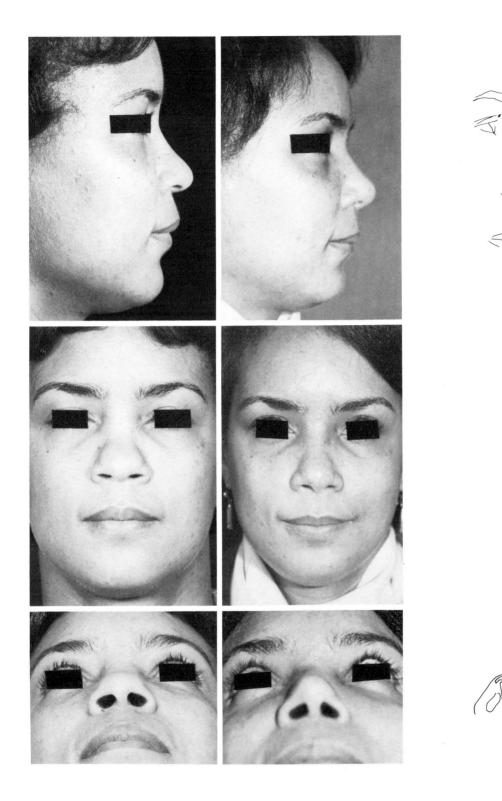

15. LARGE, SQUARE NASAL TIP

Consideration

One should take into account:

- The projection of the tip which may or may not require resection of the domes.
- The height of the domes whose reduction involves a diminution of the width by weakening.
- The width of the dome which, in the case of parallel incisions, diminishes at the expense of a slight increase in the projection.
- The type of skin (resection should be less in cases of thick skin).

Plan of operation

- An exteriorisation of the domes which permits staggered or parallel incisions.
— When the projection of the nasal tip is not increased (Fig. 5.25):
  - Reduction of the height of the domes and
  - Parallel or, better, staggered incisions, without piercing the restibular skin.
— If the projection of the nasal tip is significant:
  - A resection of the domes expending variably onto the mesial crura which are brought together.
- In cases of skin of some thickness: taping of the tip of the nose with adhesive strips at night for 30–45 days.

Fig. 5.25 Square tip, discreet hump, weakness of the middle cartilaginous third, thin skin.
— Moderate subperiosteal undermining.
— Extramucosal dissection.
— Triangular shortening (4 mm anteriorly).
— Tip:
   • Major reduction of the height of the lateral crura (height of remaining cartilage: 3 mm)
   • Exteriorisation of the domes and parallel incisions
   • High suture of the mesial crura bringing them back to back.
— Bridge: moderate lowering of the osseous hump with a rasp.
— No lateral osteotomy.
— Cartilage grafts over the middle third of the pyramid: two fragments of lateral crus are placed on each side of the septum; two fragments of crushed cartilage are placed over the superficial surface of the triangular cartilages.
— A slight augmentation of projection is obtained.
— The osseous bridge continues normally into the widened cartilaginous bridge.

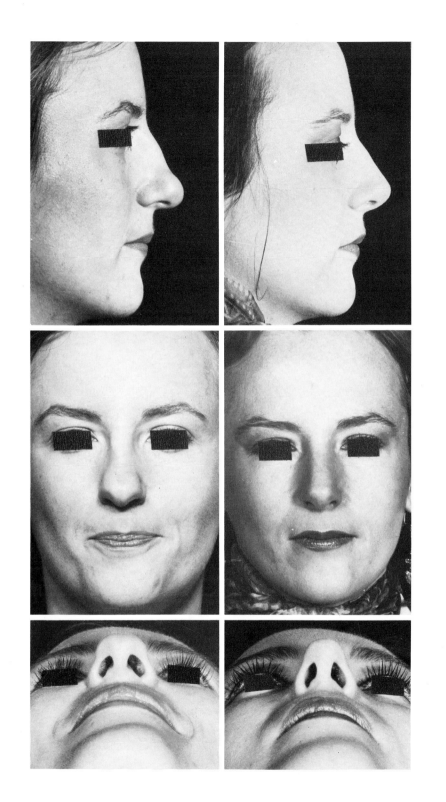

16. ULTRA-PROJECTING NASAL TIP

Considerations

One should take into account:

• The projection of the nasal bridge: after reduction of the kyphosis, the tip of the nose seems more projecting: after a cartilage graft over a receding bridge, the tip seems less large

• The skin: a thick skin calls for more conservative cartilage resections

• A cutaneous depression in the posterior portion of the nasal ala which contraindicates a resection of the tail of the lateral crura.

The more conservative concepts of nasal plastic surgery explain why cartilaginous resections carried out at the nasal tip can be less extensive.

Plan of operation

• A transfixing incision as for as the nasal spine which entails a slight loss of projection.

• A resection of the cartilaginous domes encroaching on the mesial crura to an extent dependent on the lowering desired. An excess of cutaneous lining can be reduced by undermining the vestibular skin projecting beyond the ends of the cartilage.

• In the case of thick skin, the reduction of the projection should be conservative; one can advise the use of strips of adhesive tape at night in the supra-apical area.

• A resection of the base of the nostril alae constitutes a complementary manoeuvre which is very often necessary. This resection should be carried out particularly in the outer cutaneous portion of the nasal ala (Figs 5.26 and 5.27).

Fig. 5.26 Very projecting tip, hollow naso-frontal angle, long alae. The marked naso-frontal depression further accentuates the projection of the nasal tip. The harmonious equilibrium is obtained by a lowering of the tip and filling-in of the naso-frontal angle.

— Correction of a deviation by resection of the inferior septal border.
— Exteriorisation of the domes and resections carried out particularly on the mesial crura (5 mm). The ends of the cartilages are rounded off.
— Very moderate reduction of the osseous bridge (with a rasp) and of the cartilaginous bridge.
— Filling-in of the naso-frontal angle with three superimposed fragments of the lateral crura sutured together.
— No osteotomy.
— Alae: resection largely lateral (4 mm).

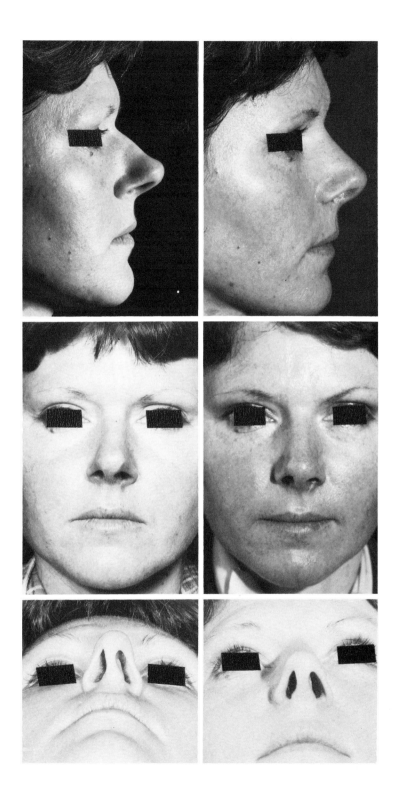

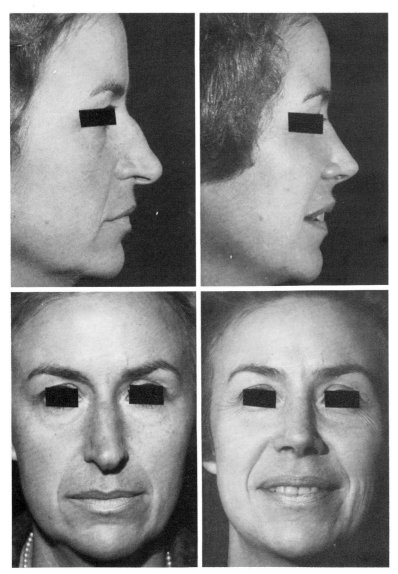
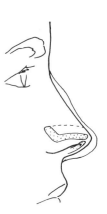

Fig. 5.27   Projecting tip, long nose, discrete hump, thin skin.

— Resection of the domes and triangular resection with an anterior base of the inferior border of mesial crura.
— Triangular shortening (5 mm anteriorly).
— Resection of the osseous hump. Lateral osteotomies.

17. DISCRETE HUMP

Getting rid of a discrete hump may seem simple; it is so when it is an isolated condition. In fact, is it often necessary to reduce, in a conservative fashion, the lateral crura, and to carry out a lateral osteotomy.

Considerations

One should take into account:

- The correction to be performed onto the root (excessively hollowed or overly projecting)
- The width of the bridge
- The projection of the tip, and a hypertrophy of the alar cartilages.

Plan of operation

- In the case of a root which is overly hollowed, after resection of the hump, a cartilage graft on the bridge extending superiorly to the root (sometimes preceded by a slight rasping) (Fig. 5.26)
- In the case of a projecting root (Fig. 5.28): a resection of the hump encroaching onto the root.
- In the case of a wide bridge:
— either a greater resection of the hump followed by reinsertion
— or a rasping (see Fig. 3.5)
— but in both cases, a lateral osteotomy with resection of the osseous corners permitting narrowing.
- In the case of a narrow bridge, one can sometimes dispense with the lateral osteotomies after rasping the hump.

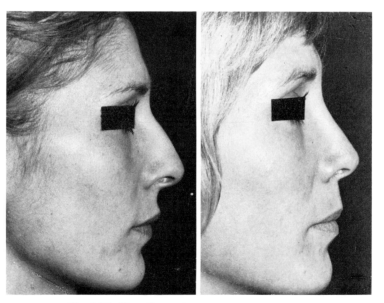

Fig. 5.28   Very discrete hump.
- High intracartilaginous incision.
- Minimal undermining.
- Reduction of the hump with a rasp.
- Very moderate reduction of the cartilaginous bridge.
- Triangular shortening (3 mm anteriorly).

18. CONSERVATIVE RHINOPLASTY

This consists of carrying out limited modifications (resections or addition of cartilage).

The patient's desire for change is moderate and one must always respect this desire, unlike that of patients who wish a major transformation.

This is a more difficult operation because the margin of error is often narrow; this method thus requires greater experience.

Two types of cases are encountered:

1. *At the request of the patient*, who has a global nasal hypertrophy, moderate or localised, which calls for correction (Fig. 5.30).

2. There exist discreet defects where *the surgeon should prescribe* discreet modifications which can involve the entire nose or be localised.

Plan of operation

● An intracartilaginous incision placed low according to the reduction to be carried out on the lateral crura.

● The dorso-nasal undermining is limited to that needed for the passage of a rasp (which will be used in most cases) or for the placement of a small cartilage graft.

● The extramucosal resection is also limited to cauterisation at the level of the mucosal dihedrons.

● If there is an osteocartilaginous hump (Fig. 5.28):
— one must begin with the rasp, then
— secondarily, resect the cartilaginous hump with a scalpel or serrated scissors.

The lateral osteotomy should not be performed if the nose is of normal width, or is narrow.

In certain cases a cartilaginous addition is indicated: when the naso-frontal angle is hollow, if the bridge or the tip of the nose is slightly receding, or if the naso-labial angle is rather closed (Fig. 5.29).

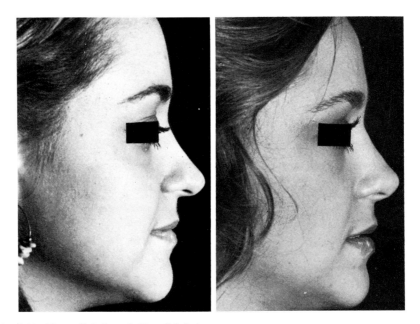

Fig. 5.29 Nose a little long, bridge slightly low.

— Triangular shortening (3 mm anteriorly).
— Septal harvesting and cartilage graft of two superimposed fragments.
— The protrusion of the ocular globes seems reduced by the elevation of the bridge by the graft.

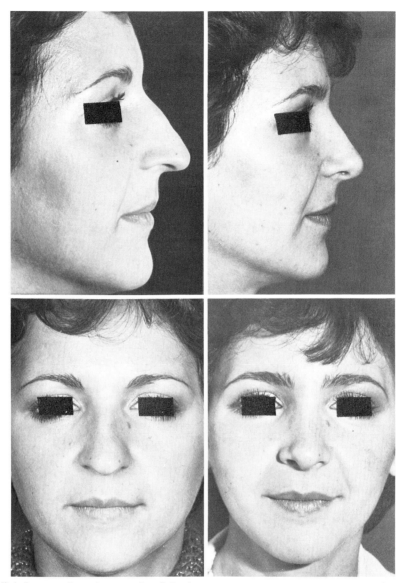

Fig. 5.30 Nose a little long, moderate hypertrophy of the tip.

— Extramucosal dissection.
— Triangular shortening (3 mm anteriorly).
— Tip: reduction of the lateral crura without section of the domes.
— Lowering of the osseous bridge with a rasp.
— Lateral osteotomy.
— Insertion of two fragments of crushed cartilage on either side of the septum, to the height of the triangular cartilages; in .
effect, the middle third of the nasal pyramid has a narrowing at this level.

19 RHINOPLASTY AND FACIAL REJUVENATION

A nose which is too long, whose tip falls toward the chin is much more frequent in the older patient. When it exists in middle-aged subjects, it accentuates the appearance of aging.

Two factors play an important role: the volume and the length of the nose. Reduction of the volume, and the elevation of the tip of the nose with opening of the naso-labial angle can have an often appreciable rejuvenating effect.

1 *Middle-aged subject* (Fig. 5.31). It is as much the reduction in volume of the nose as the shortening which plays a role here. The rhinoplasty poses fewer problems than in an older patient if the skin is in good condition.

2. *Older patient* (Fig. 5.32). Rhinoplasty is rarely requested by the older patient; when it is performed in this age group, the following particular points should be noted.

Considerations

One should take into account:

- Characteristics associated with age:
— loss of cutaneous elasticity: the cutaneous excess which is not resorbed can be significant, and require an external cutaneous excision (Peterson, *Open Flap Rhinoplasty*)
— postoperative ecchymoses are often considerable.
- The skin:
— Thick at the level of the tip or over the entire nasal pyramid: in these cases, doing nothing is often preferable
— Thin, creased with marked wrinkles, particularly over the root of the nose.
- The length of the nose.
- The extent of the hump; of a naso-frontal depression.
- The width and volume of the nose.

Plan of operation

- Always, a more conservative operation, and often an augmentation rhinoplasty.
- Hump: the reduction should be moderate and associated with a filling in of the naso-frontal angle if the root is hollow.
- Length: the shortening can be useful, on the one hand by sliding the inferior septal border between the two mesial crura, and on the other hand, by carrying out a cutaneous resection at the level of the root of the nose (generally reserved for cases with large humps, and very slack and thin skin) (see Fig. 2.65a).
- Width: osteotomies should be rare, taking account of the extent of the ecchymoses. It is preferable, in order to avoid an 'open roof', to place a graft (cartilage or a fragment of the hump) over the nasal bridge.
- The surgery of facial rejuvenation (face lifting, blephroplasty) can be associated with a very discreet manoeuvre performed on the nasal pyramid, such as shortening, rasping a small hump, or filling-in of a hollow naso-frontal angle (by a fragment of temporal fascia).

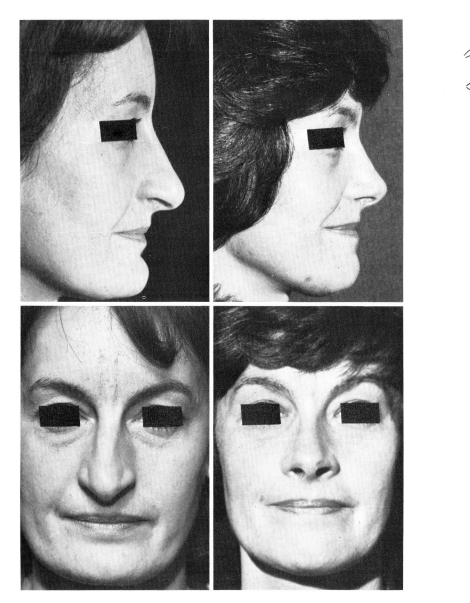

Fig. 5.31   Long nose, a discreet deviation, progenia.

— Progenia: modelling resection of the chin (through an endo-buccal approach).
— Nose:
  • Extramucosal dissection, wide subperiosteal undermining
  • Triangular mucosal shortening (5 mm anteriorly)
  • Triangular cartilaginous shortening (3 mm anteriorly)
  • Reduction of the lateral crura without section of the domes (through a contralateral approach), height of remaining cartilage: 3 mm
  • Correction of a septal deviation (by resection of the inferior septal border and the osseous septal base on the left side); lateral osteotomies
  • Insertion of septum between the two mesial crura secured by two transfixing sutures).

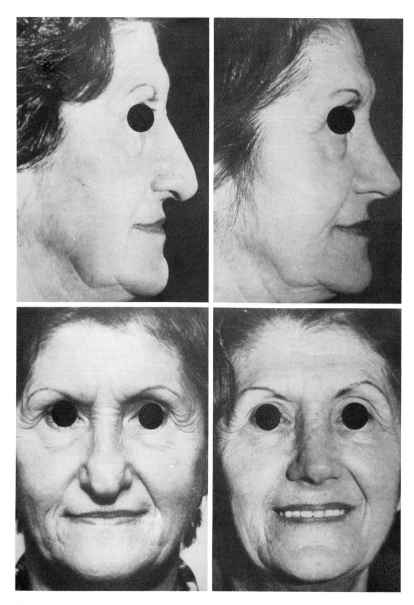

Fig. 5.32   Long nose, falling and asymmetrical tip, thin skin.

— Extramucosal dissection.
— Triangular shortening anteriorly (5 mm), resection 2 mm greater on the mucosa.
— Tip: exteriorisation of the domes and resection of the large height of the lateral crura without section of the domes.
— Resection of the osteocartilaginous hump (lowering by 2 mm).
— Osteotomy in a 'ascending curve'.
— Insertion in front of the mesial crura of a lateral fragment of the osseous hump, and insertion of the inferior septal border between the two mesial crura.

20. NOSE AND CHIN

Anomalies of the chin are most often revealed during a consultation for a rhinoplasty. They are more or less pronounced and often unrecognised by the patient. The harmony of the face requires that the correction of the chin be carried out at the same operative session as the rhinoplasty. When treatment of the retrogenia (in the great majority of cases, this is a retrogenia) is envisaged, it is sometimes useful to have a lateral film to study the anomaly more precisely, and determine the treatment which it requires.

Considerations

One should take into account:

• The extent of the retrogenia, or anomaly in the height of the lower facial third: diminished with a very marked mento-labial fold, or increased with a disappearance of the mento-labial crease, labial malocclusion at rest and an anterior open bite.
• An asymmetry.
• Problems of dental articulation for which surgery is sometimes indicated.
• A large nasal kyphosis: the hump removed in a piece can be reinserted at the level of the chin.
• The extent of the retrogenia in relation to the nasal deformity. In certain cases, improvement of the profile depends particularly on the correction of the retrogenia. When the patient does not accept this correction, one must sometimes refuse to carry out the nasal correction which would risk making more evident the receding chin.
• The desires of the patient concerning the approach, cutaneous or mucosal, and the treatment itself — a chin implant or an osteotomy.

Plan of operation

• In cases of mild retrogenia:
— Either a silicon implant (Fig. 5.33)
— Or an insertion of cartilaginous fragments or of the 'stripped' and remodelled nasal hump (Fig. 5.34).
• The approach may be external through (submental incision): the advantage here is to avoid the temporary stiffness of the lip which is seen after the endobuccal approach.
• In cases of more important retrogenia, and of anomalies in the height of the lower jaw region or an asymmetry, a suprabasilar osteotomy of the chin remains the treatment of choice, permitting (Figs. 5.35 and 5.36, see also Fig. 5.23):
— Regulation of the degree of projection of the chin
— Reduction of the height by osseous resections or overlapping of the lower fragment
— Increasing height by interposing a bone graft or modifying the direction of the osteotomy line
— Correction of an asymmetry.

Technical points

• One should conserve the median posterior muscular insertions, which has the advantage of creating a stretching of the submental region, as well as providing good vascularisation to the displaced bony fragment which is essentially cortical.
• The osteotomy line should be extended sufficiently posteriorly to obtain a good profile.
• Three wire osteosyntheses are used to maintain the correction.

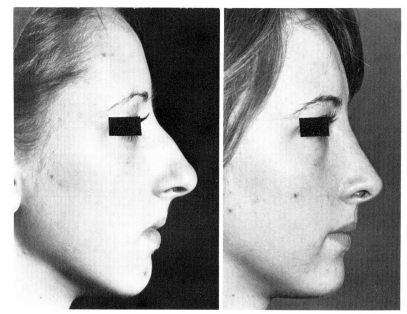

Fig. 5.33 Discreet retrogenia.

— Chin: correction by insertion of a silicone prosthesis (mucosal approach).
— Nose:
  • Rectangular shortening (3 mm anteriorly)
  • Reduction of the nasal spine
  • Tip: reduction of the height of the lateral crura
  • Resection of the osteocartilaginous hump with an osteotome
  • Lateral osteotomy in an 'ascending curve'
  • Besides the chin, the improvement is particularly noticeable in the upper lip and the naso-labial angle.

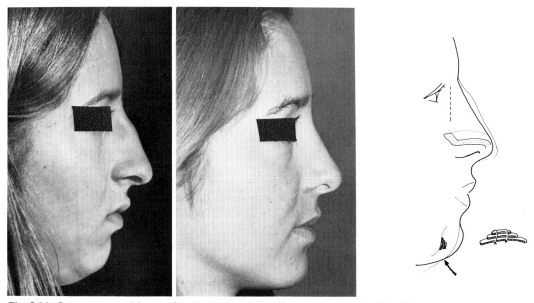

Fig. 5.34 Long nose, nasal hump of moderate size, large falling tip, retrogenia, thin skin.

— Creation of a pre-periosteal pocket in the chin through a cutaneous submental approach (incision 1.5 cm long).
— Intracartilaginous incision, moderate subperiosteal undermining.
  • Extramucosal dissection
  • Tip: resection of the superior excess of the lateral crura and of the domes, without section of the domes
  • Triangular shortening (2 mm posteriorly, 4 mm anteriorly), and discreet reduction of the nasal spine
  • Resection of the osteocartilaginous hump in a monobloc
  • Lateral osteotomies
  • Correction of a posterior septal deviation permitting the harvesting of a large amount of cartilage.
— Insertion over the chin of the hump and of cartilaginous fragments placed in three layers; suture in two planes.

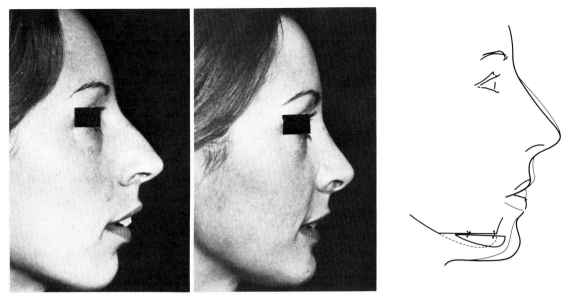

Fig. 5.35 Profiloplasty.

— Supra-basilar osteotomy of the chin through an endobuccal incision, with a 9 mm anterior sliding. An osteosynthesis with three 0.4 mm wires

— Rhinoplasty at the same operative stage (a correction of the maxillary alveolar protrusion had been carried out four months previously).

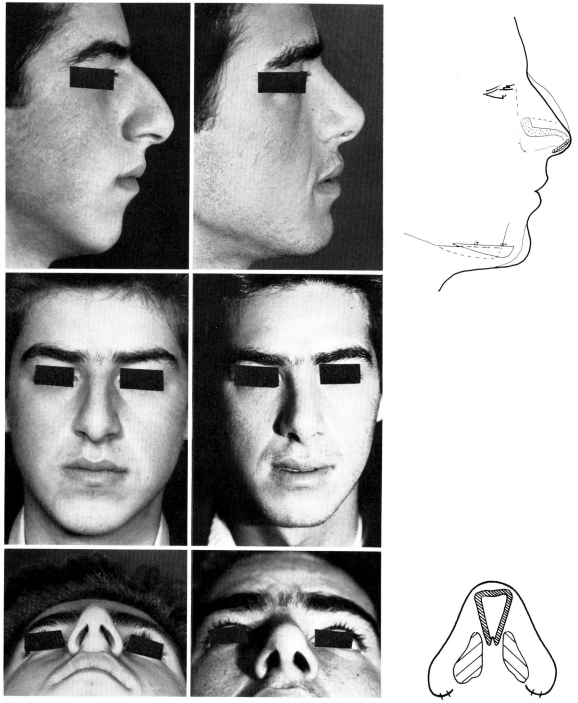

Fig. 5.36 Large nose with projecting root, osseous and cartilaginous hump, short columella, skin a little thick, retrogenia. The reduction of the extensive cartilaginous hump, and of the projecting nasal spine, caused a lowering of the nasal tip which was compensated for by a graft.

— Chin: supra-basilar osteotomy with overlapping (9 mm advancement). Osteosynthesis with three wires.
— Tip: exposure of the cartilages by a marginal incision, reduction of the height of the lateral crura; resection of the hump with an osteotome with hollowing of the root. Moderate reduction of the nasal spine. Septal harvesting: and reinforcement of the projection of the tip of the nose by triangular grafts (Sheen) over two thicknesses (fragments of the hump and a cartilage fragment placed beneath). Low lateral osteotomies. Resection of the osseous 'corners'. Reduction of the alae (3 mm).

BIBLIOGRAPHY

Aiach G 1971 Nez déviés. Gaz. Méd. France, 78: 15

Aiach G 1981 Technique d'exposition des cartilages alaires avec < anse de seau > par voie rétrograde et controlatérale. Ann. Chir. Plast., XXVI 3: 257–270

Aiach G 1982 Modifications de l'angle naso-labial au cours des rhinoplasties. Ann. Chir. Plast., XXVI 2: 137–143

Aiach G, Gomulinski L 1982 Résection contrôlée de la bosse nasale osseuse au niveau de l'angle naso-frontal. Ann. Chir. Plast., XXVII 3: 226–231

Aiach G 1974 Intérêt d'une dissection extra-muqueuse dans le traitement de certaines sténoses vestibulaires. Ann. Chir. Plast. 19 3: 273–276

Aiach G 1974 Profiloplasties: ostéotomies maxillaires supérieures et rhinoplasties. Ann. Oto-laryngol. 91 6: 341–346

Aiach G 1988 Les augmentations mentonnières (p. 119–130). Le Menton, Ed. Masson

Anderson J 1966 A new approach to rhinoplasty. Trans. Amer. Acad. Ophthalmol. Oto-laryngol. 70: 183–192

Anderson J R, Russel Ries W 1986 Rhinoplasty. Emphasising the external approach. Thieme Verlag, Stuttgart, New York

Anderson J R, Rubin W 1958 Retrograde intra-mucosal hump removal in rhinoplasty. Arch. Oto-Laryngol. 68: 346–350

Aubry M, Giraud J C, Levignac J, Secnechal G, Cusin L 1985 Chirurgie fonctionnelle correctrice et restauratrice du nez. La rhinoplastie. Arnette, Paris

Aubry M, Levignac J 1960 Le traitement des déformations par fracture ancienne de la pyramide nasale. Ann. O.R.L. 6: 405–422

Aubry M, Levignac J 1961 La petite et la grande histoire de la chirurgie plastique du nez. Histoire de la Médecine, 6 juin

Aufricht G 1969 Rhinoplasty and the face. Plast. Reconstr. Surg. 43 3: 219–230

Aufricht G 1976 Total concept of rhinoplasty. Symposium on Corrective Rhinoplasty 13: 70

Aufricht G 1943 A few hints and surgical details in rhinoplasty. Laryngoscope 53: 317

Bachmann W 1982 Die Funktions diagnostic der Behinderten Nasenatmung, Einführung in die Rhinomabometrie. Springer Verlag, Berlin, Heidelberg, New York

Baker D C 1980 Physiology Chapter. In: Aesthetic plastic surgery of T D, Rees W B Saunders. Philadelphia pp. 66–98

Becker O J 1958 Principles of oto-laryngologic plastic Surgery. Amer. Academy Ophtalmol. and O.R.L. Whiting Press, Rochester

Brown J B, McDowell F 1965 Plastic surgery of the nose. Thomas Springfield, Illinois

Bull T, Mackay I 1986 Alar collapse. Facial plast.; surg. 3: 266

Caronni E P 339 A new method to correct the nasolabial angle in rhinoplasty. Plast. Reconstr. Surg. 50: 4

Caronni E 1976 Secondary rhinoplasty. In: Trans. Internat. Cong. VI Plast. Rec. Surg. Masson, Paris pp. 490–495

Champy M 1969 A propos de la chirurgie nasale fonctionnelle et correctrice. Ann. Chir. Plast. 14: 145–152

Champy M 1968 La Septorhinoplastie. Strasbourg Méd. 19: 963–971

Cinelli J A 1958 Correction of combinated elongated nose and recessed naso-labial angle. Plast. Reconstr. Surg. 21–139

Cole P 1953 Further observations on the conditionning of respiratory air. J. Laryngol. 67: 669

Constantian M B 1985 Grafting the projecting nasal tip. Ann. Plast. Surg. 14: 391

Constantian M B 1984 Towards refinement in rhinoplasty. Plast. Reconstr. Surg. 74: 19

Constantian M B 1987 A model for planning rhinoplasty. Plast. Reconstr. Surg. 79: 3

Converse J M 1968 Reconstructive plastic surgery 2. Philadelphia W B Saunders

Converse J M 1950 Corrective surgery of nasal deviations. Arch. Oto-laryngol. 52: 671

Converse J M 1976 Symposium on corrective rhinoplasty. The Mosby Company, St Louis p. 223

Cornette de Saint-Cyr B, Guerin Surville H, Nicoletis G 1981 Agrandissement de l'orifice piriforme. Ann. Chir. Plast. 26: 276–279

Cottle M H 1954 Nasal roof repair and hump removal. A.M.A. Arch Laryngol. 60: 4, p. 408–414

Cottle M H 1955 The structure and function of the nasal vestibule. Arch. Oto-laryngol. 62: 173

Cottle M H 1960 Concepts of nasal physiology as related to corrective nasal surgery. Arch. Oto-laryngol. 72: 11

Cottle M H 1954 Nasal roof repair and hump removal. Arch. Oto-laryngol. 60: 480

Courtiss E H, Goldwyn R 1983 The effects of nasal surgery on airflow. Plast. Reconstr. Surg. 72: 1

Daniel R K, Lessard M L 1984 Rhinoplasty: a graded aesthetic-anatomical approach. Ann. Plast. Surg. 13: 436

Daniel R K, Ethier R 1987 Rhinoplasty, a CT scan analysis. Plast. Reconstr. Surg. 80: 2, 175

Delaire J The potential role of facial muscles in monitoring maxillary growth and morphogenesis. In: Carlson D S, McNamara J Jr (eds) Muscle adaptation in the cranio facial region. Monograph No 8, Center of Human growth and development. The University of Michigan. Ann. Arbor, Michigan

Delaire J 1978 L'analyse architecturale et structure cranio-faciale. Rev. Stomatol. 1: 1

Denecke H J, Meyer R 1964 Plastiche Operationen and Kopf und Hals. Springer Verlag, Berlin, Gottingen, Heidelberg

Farkas L G 1981 Anthropometry of the head and face in medicine. Elsevier New York p 52

Fombeur J P, Geneviève J P 1976 Correction des rétractions alaires post-opératoires par dissection sous-muqueuse et greffe cartilagineuse libre. Société de Laryngologie des Hôpitaux de Paris. Séance du 15 déc. 1975. Ann. Otolaryngol 93: 9, 640–643

Fry H 1967 Nasal skeletal trauma and the interlocked stresses of the nasal septal cartilage. Br. J. Plast. Swig. 20: 146

Fred G B 1955 Role of depressor septi nasi muscle in rhinoplasty. A.H.A. Arch. Orto-laryngol. 62: 1, 37–41

Gibson T, Curran R C, Davis R B 1957 The survival of living homograft cartilage in man. Transplantation Bulletin 4: 105

Goldwyn R M 1975 Aesthetic Surgery trouble. How to avoid it and how to treat it. Edited by Eugene H. Courtiss. Patient Selection: the importance of being cautious. C V. Mosby Compagny

169

Gomulinski L 1982 La traduction morphologique des déformations septales. Leur correction au cours des rhinoplasties complexes. Ann. Chir. Plast. XXVII 4: 343

Gorney M 1976 The septum in rhinoplasty: form and function. Symposium on corrective rhinoplasty. The C. V. Mosby Company, Saint-Louis, pp. 180–191

Grignon J L 1963 Les échecs des rhinoplasties. Ann. Oto-rhino-laryngol. 80: 51

Guerreros Santos J 1973 Cosmetic repair of acute columellar lip angle. Plast. Reconstr. Surg. 52 3: 246

Guerreros Santos J 1984 Temporo parietal free fascia grafts in rhinoplasty. Plast. Reconstr., Surg. 74: 465

Gunter J P, Rohrich R J 1987 External approach for secondary rhinoplasty. Plast. Reconstr. Surg. 80: 2

Gunter J P 1987 Tip rhinoplasty: a personal approach. Facial Plast Surg 4: 263

Gruber R P 1988 Open rhinoplasty. Clin. Plast. Surg. 15: 95

Hagege J C, Pollet J 1976 Le dogme du dôme. Ann Chir. Plast. XXI 3: 215

Hinderer K H 1971 Fundamentals of anatomy and surgery of the nose. Aesculapius, Birmingham

Hinderer K H 1977 Correction of deformities of the base of the nose. Plast Rec. Surg. Face and Neck. Proc. Second Internat. Symp. Vol. 1°, Grune and Stratton, San. Francisco, New York, London

Jeppesen F 1986 Septo and rhinoplasty. Munksgaard, Copenhagen

Jost G, Meresse B, Torossian F 1973 Etude de la jonction entre les cartilages latéraux du nez. Ann. Chir. Plast. 18: 175

Jost G 1975 Atlas de chirurgie esthétique plastique. Masson, Paris

Jost G, Oulie J, Hadjean E 1973 De l'opportunité de la réinclusion d'un fragment de bosse dans la correction des nez hypertrophiques. Ann. Chir. Plast. 18 2: 175

Juri J, Juri C, Colnago A 1980 Implants and grafts in secondary rhinodeformities. Aesthetic Plast. Surg. 4 2: 135

Juri J, Juri C, Elias J C 1979 Ear cartilage grafts to the nose. Plast. Reconstr. Surg. 63: 377

Kawamoto H 1982 Reduction mentoplasty: discussion. Plast. Reconstr. Surg. 70: 151

Kayle B L 1983 The onlay graft for nasal tip projection (discussion). Plast. Reconstr. Surg. 71: 36

Konno A 1969 Airflow and resistance in the nasal cavity J. Oto-laryngol. Jap. 72: 36

Le Pesteur J. Firmin F 1977 Réflexions sur l'auvent cartilagineux nasal. Ann. Chir. Plast. 22: 1

Le Pesteur J S, Sarazin, Tristan H 1976 La xérographie. Intérêt en rhinoplastie et en chirurgie maxillo-faciale. Ann. Chir. Plast. 21: 2

Levignac J 1958 Des petits et des gros ennuis dans la rhinoplastie. De la maniére de s'en sortir ou de les éviter. Ann. O.R.L.-T. 75 7–8: 560

Levignac J 1959 Greffes et implants, greffes ou implants dans la réparation du soutien nasal après enfoncement. Ann. Oto-rhino. 9: 764

Levignac J 1988 Le menton. Masson, Paris 1988

Levignac J, Chalaye J C, Mathe E, Riu R 1983 Nasal morphology and its relation to orificial musculature. Trans. VIII Congress I.P.R.S. Montréal

Levignac J 1988 Construction de la face. Esthétique et perception. Dysrythmies morphologiques et eurythmie. Ann. Chir. Plast. 33: 1

Lewis J R 1974 Atlas of aesthetic plastic surgery. Little Brown and Company, Boston

Mahe E, Gamblin J 1974 Le muscle dépresseur de la pointe. Ann. Chir. Plast. 19 3: 257

Meyer R 1988 Secondary and functional rhinoplasty. The difficult nose. Grune and Stratton New York

McKinney P, Shively R 1979 Straightening the twisted nose. Plast. Reconstr. Surg. 64: 176

McKinney P 1978 Nasal type grafts with invited comment by Thomas D. Rees. Ann. Plast. Surgery 1 2: 177

McKinney P, Stalnecker M 1983 Surgery for the bulbous nasal tip, Ann Plast Surg 11: 1060

McKinney P 1978 Nasal tip cartilage grafts. Ann. Plast. Surg. 1: 177

Mackay J S 1979 'Measurement of nasal, airflow and resistence' Jour. Royal Soc. Med. 72: 852

Micheli Pellegrini V 1975 Cause d'insuccesso nella chirugica estetica del naso. Revis. Ita. Chir. Plast., VII: 41

Micheli Pellegrini V 1985 Il naso torto. Garangola, Padua

Millard D R Jr 1972 Versatility of the chondro-mucosal flap in the nasal vestibule. P.R.S. 50: 580

Millard D R Jr 1967 Alar magin sculpturing. Plast. Reconstr. Surg. 40: 4

Millard D R Jr 1960 External excisions in rhinoplasty. Br. J. Plast. Surg. 12: 340

Monteil J P 1985 Physiologie nasale. Ann. Chir. Plast. XXX: 2

Muhlbauer W 1986 Profil rhinoplasty. Handchir. Mikrochir. Plast. Chir. 18: 90

Negus V E 1958 The comparative anatomy and physiology of the nose and paranasal sinuses. London-E., Livingstone

Natvig P, Sether A, Gingrass R P, Gardner W D 1971 Anatomical details of the osseous-cartilaginous framework of the nose. Plast. Reconstr. Surg. 48 6: 528

Ortiz Oscoy L 1981 The use of cartilage graft in primary aesthetic rhinoplasties. Plast. Reconst. Surg. 67 5: 597

Ortiz Monasterio F, Olmedo A 1977 Rhinoplasty on the Mestizo nose. Clin. Plast. Surg. 4: 89

Oulie J 1976 The high radix of the nose. Sixth International Congress of Plastic and Reconstructive Surgery, 483

Peck G C 1983 The onlay graft for nasal tip projection. Plast. Reconstr. Surg. 71 1: 27

Peck G C 1984 Techniques in aesthetic rhinoplasty. George Thieme Verlag, Stuttgart, New York

Peer L A 1941 The fate of autogenous septal cartilage after transplantation in human tissue. Arch. Oto-laryngol. 34: 697

Peer L A 1955 Transplantation of tissues, Vol. 1. Williams and Wilkins, Baltimore

Pech A, Cannoni M 1969 Anatomie chirurgicale du nez. Cahiers d'O.R.L. 4 1: 63

Pensler J, Mac Carthey J G 1985 The calvarial donor site: an anatomic study in cadavers. Plast Reconstr. Surg. 75 7: 646

Peterson R A 1976 Open flap rhinoplasty. Symposium on corrective rhinoplasty. The C.V. Mosby Company, St-Louis

Piotti F 1981 Secondary rhinoplasty. Aesth. Plast. Surg. 5 3: 259

Piotti F, Mascetti M, Gambaro, Velasco M A 1979 La deformazione postraumatica de la piramide nasale Min. Oto-rin 29: 93

Planas J 1977 The twisted nose. Clin Plast Surg 4: 55

Planas J 1964 Total extirpation of the septum. Trans 3° Internat. Cong. Plast. Surg. 538–545, 66 Excerpta Medica

Planas H 1977 The twisted nose. Clin. Plast. Surg. 4: 55

Pollet J 1972 Utilisation des exérèses ostéo-cartilagineuses au cours des rhinoplasties. Ann. Chir. Plast. 2

Pollet J, Baudelot S 1976 Séquelles de la chirurgie esthétique de la base du nez. Ann. Chir. Plast. 12 3: 185

Ponti L 1969 Surgery of the nasal tip. A modification of the Goldman technique. Proc 9th. Internat. Cong. Otorhynolaryng., México, 1969 (Exerc. Méd.) Internat. Cong. Sérics 206: 698

Portmann M et al 1983 Nez et face. Vol 2. Masson, Paris

Powell N, Humphreys B 1984 Proportions of the aesthetic face. Thieme Verlag, Stuttgart, New York

Proetz A W 1953 Respiratory air currents and their clinical aspects. J. Laryngol. 67: 1

Rees Th 1980 Aesthetic Plastic Surgery, Vol. 1. W B Saunders Company, Philadelphia

Reich J 1983 The application of dermis graft in deformities of the nose. Plast. Reconstr. Surg. 71 6: 772

Rethi A 1934 Operation to shorten an excessively long nose. Rev. Chir. Plast. 2: 85

Riu R 1980 Considérations sur la rhinorhéographie. Ann. O.R.L. Belge 34: 131

Riu R 1974 La rhinorhéographie dans la morphologie du nez et les septo-rhinoplasties. Ann. Chir. Plast. XIX 3: 181

Robin J L 1979 Extra-mucosal method in rhinoplasty. Aesth. Plast. Surg 3: 171

Rogers B O 1969 The importance of 'delay' in timing secondary and tertiary correction of post rhinoplastic deformities. In: Transaction of the Fourth International Congress of Plastic and Reconstructive Surgery, 1967, Excerpta Medica Foundation, Amsterdam, p. 1065

Safian J 1958 Fact and fallacy in rhinoplasty surgery. Br. J. Plast. Surg. 11: 52

Senechal J, Qulie J, Neveu Anatomie de la racine du nez. Cahiers O.R.L. 79: 12

Senechal G 1968 Un nouveau procédé de greffe osseuse dans le traitement des ensellures nasales. Ann. Chir. Plast, 13 3: 167

Sheen J H Spreader graft: a method of reconstructing the roof of the middle nasal vault following rhinoplasty. Plast. Reconstr. Surg. 73 2: 230

Sheen J H 1975 Achieving more nasal tip projection by use of small autogenous vomer or septal cartilage graft. Plast. Reconstr. Surg. 35: 211

Sheen J H 1978 Aesthetic rhinoplasty. The C.V. Mosby Company, St-Louis

Skoog T 1966 A method of hump reduction in rhinoplasty. Arch. Oto-laryngol. 83: 238

Stoksted P, Gutierrez C 1981 Obtaining a gentle contour to the columella by modifying the maxillary spine. Plast. Reconstr. Surg. 68 5: 689

Tamerin J A 1971 Five most important points in a reduction rhinoplasty. Plast. Reconstr. Surg. 48 3: 214

Tardy M E, Younger, Key M, Chang E 1987 The overprojecting tip. Anatomic variations and targeted solutions. Facial Plast. Surg. 4: 327

Tardy M E Jr Micro-osteotomies in rhinoplasty. Facial Plast. Surg. 1 2: 137

Tessier P 1958 Chirurgie réparatrice et morphologique du nez. Rev. du Praticien, 8 27: 3085

Tessier P 1968 La rhinoplastie esthétique. G.M. de France 75: 28

Tessier P 1982 Autogenous bone grafts taken from the calvarium for facial and cranial applications. Symposium on maxillo facial surgery. Clinics in plastic surgery 9: 4

Tisserand J 1984 La valve nasale. Thèse Médecine Nancy, 12 décembre

Tisserand J, Wayoff M 1986 La valve nasale. Les cahiers d'O.R.L. 21 4: 241 La Simarre, Tours

Tisserand J, Wayoff M 1986 La valve nasale. Arquivos portugueses de O.R.L 1: 5

Tulasne J F, Raulo Y 1981 Exceàs vertical antérieur de l'étage inférieur de la face et génioplastie. Ann. Chir. Plast. 26 4: 332

Vilar-Sancho B 1980 Secondary Rhinoplasty for correction of unfavourable results due to nasal septum. Trans of the VII Internat. Congress of Plast. Recons. Surgery Cartgraf. Sao Paulo

Walter C 1966 Die Anwendung der sogenannten Composite grafts in der plastichen Chirurgie im Hals-Nasen-Ohrenbereich. HNO Wegw. 14: 200

Walter C 1969 Composite grafts in nasal surgery Arch. Otolaryng. 90: 622

Walter C 1976 Plastische und wieder-herstellende Chirurgie zum thema; Nasen Flügelkollaps. Z Laryngol. Rhinol. 55: 447

Wayoff M, Friot J M, Chobaut J C 1977 Réflexions sur la rhinoplastie fonctionnelle. Ann. Méd., Nancy

Webster G V 1973 Skin excisions in reduction rhinoplasty. Plast. Reconstr. Surg. 51 3: 289

Willemot J 1970 Le rôle de la cloison dans la chirurgie correctrice du nez. Int. Rhinol. 8 2: 133

Willemot J 1966 L'examen du patient avant rhinoplastie corrective. Congrès Français d'Oto-Rhino-Laryngologie 63: 277

Zelnik J, Ruedi P, Gingrass R 1979 Anatomy of the alar cartilage. Plast. Reconstr. Surg. 64 5: 650

Zide B M Nasal anatomy: the muscles and tip sensation.

Index